THE

EPIDEMIC

THAT

NEVER WAS

FOREWORD

BY

DAVID A.

HAMBURG

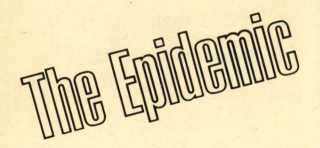

The Epidemic

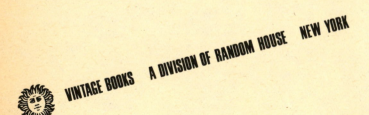

VINTAGE BOOKS   A DIVISION OF RANDOM HOUSE   NEW YORK

Books by Richard E. Neustadt

Alliance Politics

Presidential Power

Books by Harvey V. Fineberg

Clinical Decision Analysis (co-author)

RICHARD E.

NEUSTADT

AND

HARVEY V.

FINEBERG

That Never Was

POLICY-MAKING

AND THE

SWINE FLU

SCARE

Vintage Books Edition, January 1983
First Edition
Copyright © 1982 by Richard E. Neustadt and Harvey V. Fineberg
Foreword by David A. Hamburg
All rights reserved under International and
Pan-American Copyright Conventions.
Published in the United States by Random
House, Inc., New York, and simultaneously
in Canada by Random House of Canada
Limited, Toronto.

Library of Congress Cataloging in Publication Data
Neustadt, Richard E.
The epidemic that never was.
Rev. ed. of: The swine flu affair. 1978.
Bibliography: p.
Includes index.
1. Swine influenza—United States—Preventive inoculation.
2. Medical policy—United States.
I. Fineberg, Harvey V. II. Title.
RA644.I6N48 1982   353.0077'6   82–40023
ISBN 0–394–71147–5   AACR2

Manufactured in the United States of America

To Bert and Mary

FOREWORD TO THIS EDITION

On the evening of February 3, 1977, I was talking with Joseph Califano, then Secretary of the Department of Health, Education and Welfare, about issues in health policy that would be faced by the new Administration in which he had just come to office. The wide-ranging discussion was interrupted when Califano said he faced a crisis and asked my immediate help. The crisis had to do with an outbreak of influenza in Florida which was related to the swine flu immunization problem. The country had just gone through a traumatic experience in which the expected epidemic of swine flu had not occurred, but instead frightening complications of the immunization had occurred in some people. Califano was faced with the problem of how to minimize the effect of the new outbreak in Florida without risking serious additional complications. The controversy about swine flu had grown so intense that it seemed to endanger other immunization activities and indeed a broader spectrum of worthwhile initiatives for the public health.

Although I was not in government, I readily agreed to Califano's request. I was serving at that time as president of the Institute of Medicine, National Academy of Sciences, and we had considerable experience in convening broadly composed, science-based groups to examine critically from many angles difficult questions affecting the health of the public. This experience was relevant to the task facing Califano, and in any event I wanted to do everything in my power to strengthen the capability of preventive approaches to major health problems in the future. So, late into that night and throughout the next few weeks I was intimately involved with Califano and his colleagues as we grappled with the immediate problem, began to think seriously about ways of increasing the public's understanding of disease prevention, and considered the nature of preventive approaches in the years ahead.

I cannot remember now whether we discussed on that first long night of February 3 the value of constructively examining the swine flu program in a scholarly way. In any event, Califano and I talked about it on several occasions. We were agreed that important lessons could be learned from objective scrutiny of the way these decisions were made. The central intent would be to improve the quality of decision-making when facing similar problems in the future. It was my view then and still is today that the swine flu decision-making situation has much in common with other high-level decisions affecting many lives that are made in stressful circumstances characterized by much complexity and ambiguity. I have been impressed with the clarification of such decision-making problems through the work of distinguished scholars coming from several disciplinary backgrounds. Among these are Graham Allison, Alexander George, Ole Holsti, Irving Janis, Howard Raiffa and the present authors. It seemed to me then and still does five years later that the swine flu decision ought not to be a matter of recrimination but rather of constructive reflection with a view to lessons for the future. The principal players in the swine flu drama were people of immense good will, high ideals, technical competence and dedication to the public good. Yet the matter turned out in a way that was disappointing to all. How could this have happened? Surely this paradox deserves careful examination, not in a polemical but rather in an analytical mode.

Califano wisely turned to Richard E. Neustadt, one of the most distinguished scholars in the field of governmental organization and high-level decision-making. Neustadt in turn wisely turned to Harvey Fineberg, an outstanding physician and a leader in the new field of medical decision analysis. Together, they brought to the task of analyzing the swine flu experience the full range of competences required to tackle the problem in depth.

To make a decision of high quality under stressful circumstances in the face of much complexity and ambiguity is a formidable task indeed. Yet the world is full of such decision problems and leaders of large institutions must face them. Nowhere are the decisions more consequential and poignant than in government.

In principle, the decision-maker must meet certain desiderata: to identify clearly the nature and scope of the decision problem, including its boundaries; to structure the problem over time; to characterize the information needed; to fill in the structure; and then to choose a preferred course of action. Put in this way, it immediately becomes clear that the requirements are very unlikely to be met by a single perspective, let alone a single brain. To fulfill these desiderata, it will almost always be necessary to bring together a variety of competences in order to get around the contours of a multifaceted problem. These decision-making processes are increasingly being made more explicit through modern analytic techniques. But these techniques, no matter how quantitative and even elegant, cannot neglect the deeply human side of the decision-making processes. To be useful in the real world they must learn to include as grist for the analytic mill an understanding of the emotions, the value conflicts and the social pressures that shape consequential decisions. This book presents a fascinating analysis of this sort, one which is useful not only in relation to the health of the public but in relation to the health of the body politic.

The authors have approached their task without rancor. They give no cavalier dismissal to the serious, well-meaning people involved in this dramatic narrative whose lives were dedicated to improving health everywhere. On the contrary, they show much respect and sensitivity to the needs and efforts of the people who shaped the drama. There is no vindictive 20/20 hindsight here. Rather, there is a searching effort to understand institutional and decision-making processes that emerge from the drama which may have considerable utility in addressing similar problems that lie ahead.

Although the entire account is absorbing and informative, I direct the reader's attention especially to the chapter entitled "Reflections." I do this because the main points crystallized in that chapter have considerable generality in addressing major problems of public health and indeed of public policy in other spheres. Let me now briefly sketch a few reasons why I find these points so valuable.

The authors direct our attention to the value of sequential decision-making. There are nodal points at which critical evidence may be assessed and subsequent decisions made accordingly. Their account makes clear the hazards of all-or-nothing, go-or-no-go, all-at-once, now-or-never decisions in complex public health matters. They challenge us to consider what kind of evidence would make us alter course in what direction. Over a broad range of problems, I doubt whether such questions are asked often enough or taken seriously enough by leaders in public policy.

The authors also make it clear that objective analysis of policy options is not in itself sufficient, valuable though these examinations can be. They emphasize the importance of anticipating implementation. What will be necessary to make a policy work? What factors need to be taken into account in future translation of policy decision into effective program? What preparation is necessary to deal with each component if the program is to be implemented wisely? Good intentions are not enough. This means that the analysis of the problem, though crucially dependent on the hardest possible science, must also venture carefully into softer science and informed judgment from multiple vantage points. Why? In order to face in advance the probable difficulties, the likelihood of major contingencies, and the cost of going wrong.

The account of the swine flu affair beautifully illustrates the powerful and pervasive character of the mass media in public health campaigns, and by clear implication in other initiatives of broad national concern. This matter has great relevance to implementation of public policy going far beyond public health interventions. One set of problems has to do with ways in which the media can get intelligible and credible information when the matters at issue are so arcane and many putative authorities are available. Moreover, the media are not a passive recipient of accurate scientific information. They tend to transform the information in ways unfamiliar to many scientists. The media have a predilection for conflict and a tendency to amplify conflict. For these reasons and more, the analysis of media behavior is increasingly important as we seek more adequate public policy.

This volume also highlights the issue of maintaining the credibility of science-based, health-oriented institutions in situations of high uncertainty. It makes us think about ways to present difficult issues candidly without arousing excessive fear, of giving facts intelligibly, of indicating limits of knowledge, of strengthening institutions to diminish serious gaps in knowledge, and of presenting comparative likelihoods for different courses of action.

Neustadt and Fineberg point to the limitations as well as the strengths of biomedical knowledge. We know a lot about living organisms generally and about the human organism specifically, and the frontiers are rapidly being pushed outward. Yet our ignorance still exceeds our knowledge. Along with zest for future insights, modesty becomes us for now. On many vital questions crucial to wise policy formulation—as in the swine flu matter—all too many things remain unknown. Authority cannot go far to substitute for evidence. Moreover, a massive, national effort of this sort requires many kinds of knowledge—basic biology, clinical medicine, public health, law, economics, psychology and more. Thus, there is great value for decision-makers in having information and advice from many high-quality sources—i.e., not only the most interested scientists, but also disinterested scientists. This latter group involves people who can readily grasp the technical issues but whose careers have been spent at some distance from the focal problem. They not only bring new information but can raise questions, challenge assumptions and call to mind fresh perspectives. Thus, a broad-based advisory group can transcend even the finest old-boy network.

Overall, the present volume strikes me as an exceedingly valuable work of scholarship on highly consequential decision-making, involving the crucial real-world conjunction of hot and cold cognitions, of quantitative analysis and clinical judgment, of objective scrutiny and human emotions—not good or evil, not victory or defeat, but the poignant dilemmas of human experience and aspiration.

The findings are all the more useful because they converge with those of other careful, systematic studies of leadership decision-making in crisis: e.g., the Cuban missile crisis, the onset of World War I and the onset of the Vietnam War. These studies taken together have important implications about decision-making for high stakes in large institutions. Such decision-makers typically operate under serious limitations: 1) incomplete information about the situation; 2) inadequate knowledge of the relation between ends and means; thus, the leader cannot predict with high confidence the consequences of choosing a given course of action; and 3) difficulty in formulating a single criterion for use in choosing the best available option. In such a setting, strategies for dealing with cognitive complexity become essential. The leader who cannot tolerate complexity is likely to be a dangerous leader. These difficult situations typically pose multiple stakes for the decision-maker that cannot readily be reconciled.

These stakes include some concept of national interest, public good, a variety of interest groups, political constituencies, and many unknown individuals whose voices are faintly heard—not to speak of the decision-maker's family and sense of worth as a person. In principle, the leader can today elicit more relevant information and more potent analytical capabilities than ever before. And we must find ways to enhance these capacities further. But as we know from troublesome experience, these potentialities for effective problem-solving often remain unfulfilled. We must learn more about ways in which the potentiality for reasonable, well-informed decision-making can actually be achieved in difficult real-life circumstances.

A major theme in the analysis both of small advisory groups and of the larger organizational context in which leaders make decisions has to do with the strong advantages of explicitly considering a wide range of alternatives, including unpleasant ones, before making a major decision. An important line of inquiry is to clarify the factors in small groups and large organizations that tend either to inhibit or to facilitate careful consideration of multiple alternatives, especially including those the decision-maker would prefer to avoid.

In 1980, the world celebrated the global eradication of smallpox, a dreadful disease. By the end of the same year, the danger of nuclear war had come close to its all-time peak. So the human capacity for good and evil now dwarfs its previous expression in all of history. All this has happened in a moment of evolutionary time—the world we have made since the Industrial Revolution and mainly within the memory of living human beings. It is the awesome task of contemporary human beings to invent solutions to problems that are largely unprecedented in the history of the species. These problems are more demanding intellectually and socially than any we have faced before. The sciences broadly conceived can help a great deal. But to be truly effective in meeting these extraordinary human predicaments, science too must transcend its traditional boundaries and achieve a level of mutual understanding, innovation and cooperation among its disciplines rarely achieved in the past. The present work is a path-breaking step in that direction.

David A. Hamburg

President
Carnegie Corporation

CONTENTS

Part Two: New Developments and Teaching

THE AUTHORS'

INTRODUCTION TO

THIS EDITION

In 1976 the United States Government tried to immunize its whole population against a threat of world epidemic from a new influenza strain called swine flu. The scale of the endeavor was unprecedented. While a qualified success by way of numbers immunized—more than 40 million in 10 weeks—this venture was also marked by controversy, delay, administrative troubles, legal complications, unforeseen medical side effects and a progressive loss of credibility for the public health authorities concerned. The threat did not materialize.

In the waning days of this endeavor a new Secretary of the then Department of Health, Education and Welfare (HEW), Joseph Califano, asked us to prepare a report for his use, reviewing the whole program in such fashion that he personally could learn from it for future reference when comparable issues reached him for decision and oversight. We agreed and gave him a report in draft form a year later, at the end of February 1978. From March to June we reviewed our draft with several key participants, a process he agreed to, and pursued some further inquiries at his request. In June we submitted our final draft; in October 1978 he had it published as a government report, *The Swine Flu Affair: Decision-Making on a Slippery Disease*.

We reproduce our report in its entirety here. The report embodied and in some respects enlarged on our initial draft, but changed neither its language nor its flavor save where we, with further information, changed our views or altered an attributed quotation to reflect its maker's memory. In thrust, tone and suggested lessons and in all the ways we tried to highlight lessons pertinent, we thought, for Califano, this version faithfully reflects the draft he read in March 1978.

Later that month Califano was quoted as telling a medical gathering that after study he had now concluded he himself or anybody else might have made the same swine flu decisions as the previous Administration had done during 1976. This cheered us mightily; this was the initial, perhaps even the chief, of the lessons we sought to convey—and a necessary preliminary to consideration of all others. Califano had come into office thinking differently: "fiasco" was the kindest word he tended to apply to those decisions at the time he asked us to review them. He had witnessed them and their results from outside as a Washington observer and a Democratic stalwart viewing Gerald Ford's Administration. Our first task was to make him see that the complexities and uncertainties of the swine flu case transcended personalities or parties. In this we feel sure we succeeded.

Our wish to make that initial point dictated the form, tone, style, sentence structure and even word choice of the report we sent Califano: we had to keep a busy and beset man *reading* while we tried to make him empathize with problems and persons he already had weighed and found wanting. He himself gave us a clue on how this might be done by asking at the outset for a "Skybolt study of swine flu." The reference was to a report on problems with the British about air-to-surface missiles which one of us had written years before for John F. Kennedy. The reading problem then had been resolved by rendering the whole report into a story told in as fast-paced and readable a fashion as the writer could contrive, with lessons conveyed by the story itself. Kennedy had read it through, and so, unknown to us, had Califano, then a young assistant to the Secretary of Defense. We took it that he liked the form, so we resolved to use it with some modifications.

In the Skybolt report, Kennedy had read about disasters to himself and his associates. This was expected, rightly it turned out, to make him sensitive to every nuance in the reading. In our report on swine flu, Califano would be reading mostly about other people's troubles, those of immediate predecessors, liable to discounting on both scores. Moreover, he would read about those others with the critical perspective of a former White House aide to Lyndon Johnson. Faced by such a reader, we thought ourselves entitled, indeed virtually required, to adopt the method of a nineteenth-century novelist: our narrative is punctuated by asides to the reader, that is to say to Califano personally. We stepped into the story, commenting by hindsight, whenever we suspected that our reader's scorn required to be curbed, or sympathy aroused, attention redirected, or indifference dispelled. These comments might have been excised from our second, published draft, but we decided not to do so. It was Califano's choice to publish our report as promptly as he did, and he asked for no changes except those reflecting any further information we acquired. We felt bound by the spirit of his choice to give the public something quite precisely comparable, editorially, to what we had first given him, including our asides. We hoped of course for other lesson-learners besides him. When we teach portions of the narrative by the case method (see Chapter 15) we find it useful to warn students against sentences that otherwise might stifle (by preempting) class discussion. With our original reader, we had no fear of stifling discussion; quite the contrary.

This edition makes no substantive changes in our text as originally published by the Government Printing Office. Since then we have encountered public health professionals who take its readability as almost a personal insult—the suggestion being, sadly, that nothing readable is serious—and our judgmental interventions as unpardonable since neither of us is an expert virologist or immunologist and one of us is medically a layman. But the lessons Califano sought to learn were managerial, not medical, at a broad, political level, not a narrow, technical one. And the way we sought to teach was by arresting his attention with a lively narrative, the nearest we could come to a vicarious experience, making our points through it as well as in addition to it. We would like to satisfy our critics but can offer no apologies for that. And while we see a few words we might usefully have altered, here and there, or room for phrases we might usefully have added, we think our report must remain what it was, infelicitous phrasing and all, a government document of given date, belonging to a certain time, open to criticism "as was." Anything else seems Orwellian.

Instead we add this preface, in an effort to be clear about our purposes and style, and three new chapters in an effort to enhance the book's utility for teaching. Chapter 14 brings up to date, through July 1981, the textual chapter on legislative and administrative legacies—where little has happened since 1978 except frustration of the plans of influenza immunologists—and the Technical Afterword, where much has been learned recently about the molecular structure and genetic composition of the influenza virus. This new knowledge is exciting and eventually may lead to more predictably effective preventives. In the meantime, influenza continues to produce surprises at a clinical and epidemiological level. It remains at least as slippery a phenomenon today at it was in 1976 or 1978.

Teaching material, a set of case studies, was what we hoped to gain when we initially accepted Califano's invitation. We began our study by assuming he would probably not wish to publish quickly a report to him planned along Skybolt lines. (The full report to Kennedy continues to be classified by order of the National Security Council staff.) But Harvard University, through which he contracted for portions of our time, does not engage in classified research. Nor would HEW then have proposed security classification for our subject. Everybody understood that in some form our study would (and should) be published. But the only form in which we had a stake when we began was a succession of self-contained pieces, each suitable as a particular assignment for a given class; in short, "cases." And we didn't much care when we got them.

This later upset some university officials, fearing lest such cases leave some things unsaid or understated for pedagogical purposes; that could well have happened. Might the excised parts of what we first gave Califano then have been deemed "classified"? The issue never arose. It was mooted by his choice to publish promptly what we gave him. Harvard's policy on classified research remained inviolate. And public access was assured without anyone's resort to the Freedom of Information Act.

The issue of public access ran deeper than we and Califano knew when we embarked upon a "Skybolt study of swine flu." This was confirmed for us in 1979, when for a time it seemed that we might have to defend in court our claimed right as scholars to maintain the confidentiality of interviews, a right which the Supreme Court has yet to recognize. The sources for our study had been press materials and documents from governmental files, along with scores of interviews. We had assured all persons interviewed that nothing would be publicly attributed to them without their consent. When Califano chose to make our report public we had first to clear all quoted comments. When our files were subsequently sought in Federal court discovery proceedings under suits arising from the swine flu program, we decided in advance to refuse a demand for our interview notes. When the time came, the demand was not made. We appreciate the legal advice of our counsel, Floyd Abrams.

We flag the issue for anyone inclined to try a study of this sort. The precedent of Skybolt was a good one, we believe, for an executive intent on drawing lessons from experience, whether his own or his predecessor's. But domestic spheres of policy are tricky to work in terms that give the manager the intimate detail from which to learn while at the same time safeguarding the privacy of sources.

Returning to our stake in eventual teaching material, Chapter 15 notes how we and others have found ways to use the swine flu study for a variety of teaching purposes. These range far beyond public health problems, *per se*. The reconstructed story was educative for Califano—also we hope for others in HEW—and putting it together certainly was educative for us. The report is longer than the teaching cases we once imagined might emerge from our study. Still, we think the full report conveys lessons more vividly than condensed cases might have done, and anyway it can be broken into separately read parts. Also, one of our Harvard colleagues, Laurence Lynn, wishing to stress aspects that for Califano's purposes we skimped, prepared a separate case, reinterviewing in the process. It elaborates our Chapters 3 and 4 at the Assistant Secretary level in HEW, where Lynn himself served under Elliot Richardson. We include in this edition the greater part of Lynn's text, with permission, as Chapter 16. We are grateful to him for the opportunity and to the Kennedy School of Government for the permission. Mindful that our interview notes were confidential, he arranged to reinterview some of the central players. Their quoted comments usefully enlarge on those in earlier chapters. Plainly his subjects had read our report; there is no help for that.

Chapter 15 is not a teaching manual in the sense of a complete account of anybody's class procedure. It could not be that and still be printed in the same book with our text or Lynn's. But it goes far enough, we hope, to give prospective teachers a clear indication of the uses made by us and others, in what sorts of courses, for what kinds of students. New users can consult us for more detail if desired.

It is because we and others find our report useful to students, usable in teaching, that we welcomed the prospect of a new edition published by Vintage Books. We are grateful to Random House for undertaking it and to our editor, Grant Ujifusa, for seeing us through. The Government Printing Office has many virtues. But, as we are often told by disgruntled teachers and students, filling orders which do not include exact change and precise stock numbers is not one of them. Besides, we now can add to what our report offered in its earlier edition. We take pleasure in that.

The swine flu program began with a bet and ended with a happenstance. At the outset a New Jersey public health official bet the doubting chief of medicine at Fort Dix that the sickness on the base was influenza. At the end, one of the first clinicians to report Guillain-Barré syndrome in a swine flu vaccinee did so because he thought he had just heard of the association on an educational cassette tape about swine flu. The tape (Audio-Digest Foundation, Family Practice, Volume 24, Number 38) was recorded at a conference held at the University of California, Los Angeles, just as vaccinations were getting under way in

October 1976. On the tape, Dr. Paul F. Wehrle tells how difficult it is to distinguish incidental illness from true side effects:

Problems with diseases that may be confused or incorrectly interpreted as induced by the influenza vaccine I think will occupy a lot of our time and a lot of our attention. We have at any one time in the state of California somebody who is in the process of developing the Landry-Guillain-Barré-Strohl or Guillain-Barré syndrome, the paralytic episode with sensory loss and so on, just spontaneously. Usually we have no indication of anything that's setting this kind of a problem off. I can assure you, though, that if someone is developing this and receives the influenza vaccine within about thirty days of the time of onset of that illness, that this influenza vaccine will be blamed either for initiating it or for making it worse.

As we did not know when we wrote our report but have learned since, the listening clinician *mistakenly* believed that he had been alerted to a *likely* complication. He looked for it and found it and was right for the wrong reasons.

On February 8, 1979, we testified before the U.S. Senate Subcommittee on Health and Scientific Research on differences between the crash program of 1976, the nationwide effort against swine flu, and a small-scale, targeted influenza initiative Secretary Califano was attempting—unsuccessfully, as it turned out—to fund on a continuing basis. We took the opportunity to put on record an explicit judgment of the 1976 program's capacity to cope had swine flu's threat become actual, a pandemic. To quote our testimony:

. . . the crash program [achieved a] . . . dubious reputation in medical, press and governmental circles generally—save for a gallant band among its early sponsors who have lately told the press that if they had it to do over they would do the same again.

Our report, we hope, aids understanding of their genuine dilemmas and attests to their good purposes, but does not rehabilitate the program's reputation. Our readers are free to judge for themselves, and we try to provide enough evidence for that. But we judge that the program, as it actually developed and was managed, deserves its dubious standing.

Moreover, we judge that its reputation probably would be no

better now (and might be worse) had swine flu actually appeared and swept the country in the fall or winter months of 1976. This judgment is implied in our report but nowhere stated bluntly. We appreciate the opportunity to repair the omission here.

We make these judgments because the administrative aspects of the swine flu program—its machinery for implementation and adjustments, and the skills of those at work there—interacted badly with the slippery features of the disease. That interaction, we believe, was almost bound to foster adverse media reactions, medical skepticism, intergovernmental backbiting, congressional concern, and public puzzlement, leading toward a credibility gap of serious proportions between Federal authorities and those they sought to serve. Television network news, an intermediary, was itself part of the problem, one those authorities never came near resolving, and their troubles in that respect might well have dogged them through an epidemic, rendering the credibility gap worse.

We find no villains in the Federal government's officials and advisers then and think that anyone (ourselves included) might have done as they did—but we hope not twice.

These remain our sentiments. The opposite danger, of course, is that the lessons of the crash program are learned too well—too literally—producing stalemate in the face of the next out-of-routine threat from influenza. Someday there will be one.

R.E.N.
H.V.F.

Wellfleet, Massachusetts
July 1981

PART ONE

THE

ORIGINAL

REPORT

INTRODUCTION

In early February 1977, less than two weeks after taking office as Secretary of Health, Education and Welfare, I was faced with a difficult health policy decision: whether to release stocks of influenza vaccine that had been withheld after use of the vaccine was linked with the Guillain-Barré Syndrome—an often paralyzing and sometimes killing side effect.

In the fall of 1976, HEW had begun vaccinating millions of citizens in an unprecedented national influenza program—an attempt to vaccinate virtually the entire American population against swine flu, and to vaccinate high-risk persons against both swine flu and A/Victoria flu.

Two main formulations of vaccine had been produced for this nationwide immunization drive: one, monovalent—the swine flu vaccine alone; the other, bivalent—the swine flu vaccine combined with A/Victoria vaccine. But over a two-month period in the fall of 1976, use of these vaccines on millions of people had turned up a hitherto unrecognized association between flu vaccine and Guillain-Barré Syndrome. Was Guillain-Barré the result of the swine flu vaccine, the A/Victoria vaccine, or all flu vaccines? No one could be certain.

But we had to make a decision. On January 29, 1977, A/Victoria flu had erupted in a nursing home in Miami. There was the possibility that this flu could become widespread, endangering high-risk groups such as the elderly and those with chronic lung disease. If it did spread, the risks of influenza would far outweigh the risk of Guillain-Barré. But there was no way to gauge the extent of the danger; and the A/Victoria vaccine was available only in the bivalent formulation: in combination with the swine-flu vaccine. Thus, a decision to release the A/Victoria vaccine was necessarily a decision to release the swine flu vaccine.

In the end, after much debate and on the advice of the experts, I decided to release the bivalent vaccine. But in the course of making this decision, I was impressed by the enormous difficulty that a lay official has in fulfilling his responsibility to make sound, balanced judgments about complex scientifically-based public health issues. From briefing papers I had read before becoming Secretary and discussions of other issues, I knew I was soon to be faced with other difficult public health questions—ranging from setting guidelines for recombinant DNA research to issues relating to psychosurgery and sterilization—that would require a careful weighing of scientific fact, some of it speculative, with ethical and policy considerations.

As a lawyer and former special assistant to former Secretary of Defense Robert S. McNamara and President Lyndon Johnson, I had frequently faced situations with little or no initial knowledge of the complex substance of the events or subject matter involved. This swine flu situation surprised and bedeviled me, however, because I knew so little that it was difficult even to determine *the questions to ask* in an attempt to reach an intelligent decision.

During this experience—and the review of the swine flu program it occasioned—I was struck that those who might find themselves facing sensitive health policy decisions could benefit greatly from a careful study of that program.

If the swine flu experience had any lessons to teach, it was important that we learn them. If there had been mistakes or missteps—however well-intentioned—it was important to learn what they were so we might not repeat them, either in immunization policy or in other, similar decision-making contexts.

Indeed, the swine flu experience threw into sharp relief two questions that increasingly challenge officials at the high policy levels of government:

- First, how shall top lay officials, who are not themselves expert, deal with fundamental policy questions that are based, in part, on highly technical and complex expert knowledge—especially when that knowledge is speculative, or hotly debated, or when "the facts" are so uncertain? When such questions arise, with how much deference and how much skepticism should those whose business is doing things and making policy view those whose business is knowing things—the scientists and the experts?
- How should policymakers—and their expert advisers—seek to involve and to educate the public and relevant parties on such complicated and technical issues? To what extent can there be informed and robust public debate before the decision is reached?

Increasingly, the questions that Presidents, cabinet officers and other officials confront involve extraordinarily technical complexities and uncertainties: defense policy and disarmament choices involving sophisticated and expensive weapons systems, for example; health policy decisions involving subtle questions of scientific possibility and probability.

With these questions in mind, I remembered an illuminating report I had read several years ago about another problem-laden episode, the Skybolt missile affair.

President John F. Kennedy, in a difficult and controversial decision, had canceled the Skybolt missile—setting off a chain of diplomatic consequences which, to the dismay of the President and his advisers, none of them seemed to have foreseen. Somewhat shaken, President Kennedy invited Professor Richard E. Neustadt of Harvard, a renowned scholar of the Presidency and the decision-making process in government, to trace the Skybolt affair and prepare a report that might draw some lessons for future policymaking. As a newcomer to the staff of Defense Secretary McNamara in the early 1960's, I read Neustadt's report to President Kennedy. I found it a fascinating narrative—and a sobering, cautionary tale.

Now Professor Neustadt and his able colleague, Dr. Harvey V. Fineberg, at my request, have anatomized the swine flu affair —in search of lessons for the future, not of fault in the past. I asked them to give me as objective and clinical a report as they could write. This book is their report. The views and observations they express here, I should stress, are their own. I sought neither to direct nor to influence the report—only to learn from it.

Their narrative will prove enormously valuable to policy-makers in this Department facing difficult decisions in the future —and needing to steer by the light that a clear, objective history can shed upon their way. Indeed, this study can have great meaning for all citizens, within government and outside it, who are interested in the process by which large decisions are made —and who are eager to improve that process.

Joseph A. Califano, Jr.

Secretary
Department of Health,
Education, and Welfare
July 1978

LETTER OF TRANSMITTAL

Honorable JOSEPH A. CALIFANO, JR.
Secretary of Health, Education and Welfare
Washington, D.C. 20201

Dear Mr. Secretary:

We present to you our study, done at your request, of Federal decision-making on the swine flu program from March 1976 to March 1977. We include the program's legacies of policy in the year after and our own retrospective reflections, along with a technical afterword. The study's coverage runs to March 1978. The study's terms are indicated further in our foreword.

We have sought details for the sake of lessons. The search was educational for us, but that is not the point. We hope it proves useful to you.

Sincerely,

RICHARD E. NEUSTADT

HARVEY V. FINEBERG

Harvard University
June 1978

ACKNOWLEDGMENTS

Four of the principal participants in the swine flu program came to Cambridge at our invitation to review the first draft of this study. They commented freely, we listened attentively, then made what seems to us a careful judgment on each point. Whether they will agree is not for us to say. But what we can say is that we appreciate their courtesy, applaud their candor, and consider ourselves fortunate to have had their counsel.

Several Harvard colleagues and a few outside observers read and commented on chapters in draft. We are grateful to all, especially to those who offered criticism. We may not have taken it to their satisfaction, but we certainly thought about it, with benefit on almost every page.

We are grateful also to the many HEW officials who cheerfully responded to requests for files, and to the GAO officials who let us review some of their workpapers on state plans. We are grateful to still larger numbers of present and former officials from many parts of government who made themselves available for interviews. Our gratitude extends no less to persons in the private sector, scientific advisers, drug company officers, insurance executives and members of the press, both print and electronic, who let *us* interview *them*. To the Columbia Broadcasting System, which made TV transcripts available, and to Vanderbilt University, which lent us tapes, we offer thanks as well.

We have done this work part-time during the academic year 1977–78 and have been helped by two extraordinary research assistants, Thomas Kinsock of the Harvard Law School, class of 1979, and Michael Holt of the Harvard Medical School, class of 1980. Our files are extensive, our interviews many; these two know everything and can find anything. They also are severe at copy-editing, and in the realm of policy they make, we think, sophisticated judgments. We are grateful to them. And to our secretary, Sally Makacynas, goes our gratitude on behalf of our readers.

R.E.N.
H.V.F.

FOREWORD

The swine flu program of the Federal government was launched in March 1976 with a White House announcement by President Gerald R. Ford. The program was finally set aside in March 1977, when HEW Secretary Joseph A. Califano, Jr., stated influenza prospects for the coming year. These did not include swine flu. The program thus outlasted, although not for long, the Ford Administration.

The National Influenza Immunization Program, the official title for this venture, was unprecedented in intended timing and in scope among American immunization efforts. It aimed at inoculating everyone before December 1976 against a new flu strain that might conceivably become as big a killer as the flu of 1918, the worst ever. The program was funded by Congress through a $135 million appropriation, and it was later buttressed by special legislation in the field of liability. It was conducted through state health departments, with technical assistance from health agencies in HEW. Inoculations started late, October 1, 1976. They had been slowed somewhat by difficulties in deciding children's dosages and seriously stalled by liability issues. On December 16, the program was suspended to assess statistical evidence of a serious side effect. Mass immunization never started up again. As a full-scale operation, the program's life was thus not twelve months but two and a half.

The killer never came. The fact that it was feared is one of many things to show how little experts understand the flu, and thus how shaky are the health initiatives launched in its name. What influenza needs, above all, is research.

Decision-making for the swine flu program had seven leading features. To simplify somewhat, they are:

- Overconfidence by specialists in theories spun from meager evidence.
- Conviction fueled by a conjunction of some preexisting personal agendas.
- Zeal by health professionals to make their lay superiors do right.
- Premature commitment to deciding more than had to be decided.
- Failure to address uncertainties in such a way as to prepare for reconsideration.
- Insufficient questioning of scientific logic and of implementation prospects.
- Insensitivity to media relations and the long-term credibility of institutions.

These and other features are discussed and qualified below.

One thing we are convinced the program was not. Whatever the contemporary notions from outside, it wasn't party politics; President Ford wanted to protect the public health.

In the year of its formal existence from March to March, the swine flu program chalked up numbers of accomplishments which give it weight historically. In these terms it may go down as a qualified success. More than 40 million civilians were inoculated, twice the number ever reached before in one flu season. A notable surveillance system was developed, better than anything before. A serious side effect of influenza vaccination, Guillain-Barré syndrome, occasionally fatal, was tracked by that system and remains under investigation. A critical policy problem for all public health interventions and research, the problem of liability, was brought into sharp focus for the first time; it is now being addressed at policy levels both in HEW and in Congress. The flu as a disease and shots as a preventive were dramatized sufficiently so that a permanent program aimed at high-risk groups is now in view. With that comes what the influenza specialists in public health have long desired, recognition for the flu alongside polio or measles among Federally supported immunization initiatives.

While media attention focused on the troubles of the swine flu program—which were many—net effects on general public consciousness seem small. Possibly, indeed, they will turn out on balance to have been more positive than negative for public health. Swine flu may have a bad ring in public ears, but millions may have heard of flu shots for the first time. On this nobody has good information.

Yet to attentive publics in and near the Washington community, to doctors in the country's schools of medicine and public health, to professionals in print and electronic journalism, to members of Congress and the Carter Administration, also to most members of the Ford Administration, the swine flu program was once widely seen and is now overwhelmingly recalled as a "fiasco," a "disaster," or a "tragedy."

More interesting still, it was and is a trauma to the government officials most involved and to their scientific advisers. A year and more later, cheeks flush, brows furrow, voices crack.

In February 1977, as the program waned, Secretary Califano asked us to review and reconstruct it in detail for his own education. His purpose was managerial. He sought lessons for the future useful to a man in his position. He had just authorized a limited resumption of the program through the rest of the flu season for the sake of high-risk groups. His position and its problems were vivid in his mind. Lessons were what he wanted, not a history; finger-pointing did not interest him in terms of last time; his concern was with next time.

Yet as he was aware, having read a comparable report by one of us done years ago for President Kennedy, we know no better way to draw most lessons than to tell the applicable portions of the story. We began with that bias. It was only reinforced when we discovered the persistence and pervasiveness of trauma. The lessons of this program, we believe, will be obscured for relative outsiders unless they understand why it had such profound effects, *not* on the country but rather on its own participants.

That understanding is imparted best by a selective narrative.

This calls for a reconstruction of events, which we have undertaken by combining press accounts, hearings, official files, and interviews with participants, as many as we could reach during the time we had available. Our efforts still leave some participants unreached, some happenings unrepresented. We are sorry for that but time pressed. In establishing "what happened" we have sought not less than three and preferably five opinions when there were as many or more persons present. In the case of actions taken by one person we have sought both his account and the impressions of contemporary bystanders, along with written records if available. Throughout we have sought views from informed observers.

This remains a reconstruction. It cannot be "the" truth as actually experienced, for there were many truths then, all imperfectly recalled; we now select among them with the benefit of hindsight. We are surely not infallible; we seek to be responsible; the judgment is our own.

Many of our informants spoke for background only. All were offered confidentiality if they so chose. Therefore, attributed quotations from our interviews have all been checked with sources for accuracy and propriety. As cannot help but happen, checks produced some changes of memory, or concerns about good taste, or insistence on non-attribution. For quotation purposes we honor the source's preference. Readers need not fear. This does not change the substance of the story; it just makes for a little less enjoyment in the reading.

What follows is our response to the Secretary's request, written for him and for whomever else he chooses. There are ten chapters of narrative, ending in March 1977. We do not deal with everything. We deal with those things we believe can best help Califano think ahead. Chapter 11 sketches open issues in the swine flu program's wake: a national commission, liability legislation, and a new immunization initiative. These we watched while researching the earlier story. We are current through March 1978. We then stopped watching; for the last three months we have been editing. Those issues remain open but our text closed as of March, a year after the program's termination.

We conclude these chapters with our own reflections, placed in Chapter 12. They bring us to administrative issues and to realms of current policy for Russian flu and after. They bring us also to the underlying issues posed by current knowledge about influenza, and by ignorance as well. We deal here with a slippery disease. What makes it so we address in a technical afterword.

There follow five appendices. "A" is a "cast of characters" named in our narrative, and a chart of certain agency relationships. "B" is a glossary of abbreviations and "C" is a detailed chronology from January 1976 to mid-March 1977. "D" contains certain documents described in narrative chapters, and "E" offers questions useful for the next pandemic threat.

With preliminaries over we can now begin.

1

THE NEW FLU

The proximate beginning of this story is abrupt. On the East Coast of the United States, January 1976 was very cold. At Fort Dix, New Jersey, training center for Army recruits, new men fresh from civilian life got their first taste of barracks and basics. A draft of several thousand came in after New Year's Day to be instructed by a cadre back from Christmas leave. The fort had been almost emptied; now in the cold it was full again. By mid-January many men began reporting respiratory ailments. A relative handful were hospitalized. One, refusing hospitalization, went on an overnight hike and died.

After a county medical meeting on another subject, the state's chief epidemiologist bet the senior Army doctor that Fort Dix was in the midst of an influenza virus epidemic. To win, the latter sent a sample set of cultures for analysis in the state laboratory. He lost. The lab turned up several cases of flu traceable to the Victoria virus, which had been since 1968 the dominant cause of human influenza.[1] But the lab also found other cases of flu caused by a virus it could not identify. With foreboding, Dr. Martin Goldfield, the civilian epidemiologist, sent those cultures to Atlanta, to the Federal government's Center for Disease Control (CDC). A similar virus, also unidentified, was isolated from the dead man and a culture sent to CDC. In the evening of February 12, the Center's laboratory chief, Dr. Walter Dowdle, reported the result to his superiors—in four cases, including the fatality, the unknown was swine flu. At CDC this caused more concern than surprise.

Four things combined to create the concern. First, these four recruits could have been infected through human-to-human transmission. Not since the late 1920's had this form of influenza been reported in as many persons out of touch with pigs. There might have been a number of occasions unreported; no one knew. Second, for a decade after World War I a virus of this sort was believed to have been the chief cause of flu in human beings. Since then it had confined itself to pigs. Were it returning now to humans, none younger than 50 would have built up specific antibodies from previous infection. Third, the Fort Dix virus differed in both its surface proteins, termed "antigens," from the influenza virus then circulating in the human population. This difference, in expert terms an "antigenic shift," would negate any resistance carried over from exposure to the other current viruses. In 1976, it was assumed by leading experts that pandemics follow antigenic shifts as night from day.

And finally, in 1918, a pandemic of the swine flu virus, the most virulent influenza known to modern medicine, had, in a so-called "killer wave," been associated with some 20 million deaths worldwide, 500,000 here. Many were taken by bacterial pneumonia, a complication of influenza now treatable with antibiotics, but an unknown number succumbed to the flu itself. Among the hardest hit then had been able-bodied persons in their twenties and early thirties. Parents of small children died in droves. So did young men in uniform. Virulence cannot as yet be tested in the lab. Could the Fort Dix swine flu be a comparable killer? No one at CDC knew any reason to suppose it was—contrast the 1920's and the circumstances of the one death now—but still. . . .

The absence of surprise reflected expert views at that time about epidemic cycles and about the reappearance of particular types of viruses in people. It was widely thought—on rather scanty evidence—that antigenic shifts were likely about once a decade (interspersed with slighter changes, "drifts," each second or third year). There had been shifts in 1957 and in 1968, both followed by pandemics—Asian flu and Hong Kong flu respectively—and public health officials were expecting another by, say, 1978 or 1979. 1976 was close. The very day the Fort Dix cases were identified at CDC, the *New York Times* carried an Op Ed piece by Dr. Edwin D. Kilbourne, one of the country's most respected influenza specialists, extolling cycles and affirming that pandemics occur every eleven years—another one of which, he warned, was surely coming soon:

Worldwide epidemics, or pandemics, of influenza have marked the end of every decade since the 1940's—at intervals of exactly eleven years—1946, 1957, 1968. A perhaps simplistic reading of this immediate past tells us that 11 plus 1968 is 1979, and urgently suggests that those concerned with public health had best plan without further delay for an imminent natural disaster.[2]

Also, an influenza virus recycling theory was just then receiving attention, and this suggested swine-type as a likely next strain to appear. The idea was that the flu virus had a restricted antigenic repertoire and a limited number of possible forms, requiring repetition after a time period sufficient for a large new crop of vulnerable people to accumulate. The Asian flu of 1957 was thought to have resembled flu in the pandemic year of 1889. The Hong Kong flu of 1968 was thought to be like that of 1898. Swine flu, absent for 50 years, fit well enough, no surprise. The theory had been originally proposed by two doctors who wrote in 1973:

A logical sequel to the data presented and supported here would be the emergence in man of a swine-like virus about 1985–1991. . . . Regardless of one's view as to the origin of recycling of human strains of influenza, the matter of being prepared to produce swine virus vaccine rapidly should receive consideration by epidemiologists. Man has never been able to intervene effectively to prevent morbidity and mortality accompanying the emergence of a major influenza variant, but the opportunity may come soon.[3]

Though some experts were skeptical about the regularity with which previous strains might be expected to reappear, no one doubted that a swine flu virus might well re-emerge in the human population.

On February 12, alerted by preliminary lab reports, Dr. David Sencer, CDC's Director, asked a number of officials from outside his agency to join him there for a full lab report on February 14. The Army responded, as did Goldfield from New Jersey. And from two other parts of CDC's parent entity in HEW, the Public Health Service (PHS), Dr. Harry Meyer and Dr. John Seal came as a matter of course. Meyer was Director of the Bureau of Biologics (BoB) in the Food and Drug Administration; Seal was the Deputy Director of the National Institute for Allergy and Infectious Diseases (NIAID) in the National Institutes of Health. (NIAID's director left these relations to Seal.) The BoB was responsible for licensing and testing flu vaccines, the NIAID for Federally sponsored flu research. The duties of Meyer and Seal overlapped, but they were accustomed collaborators. Both were accustomed also to work closely with CDC, its labs and its state services.

Among their recent objects of collaboration had been workshops held at intervals since 1971 on how to better the quite dismal record of 1957 and of 1968 in getting vaccine to Americans ahead of a pandemic. This matter was much on Seal's mind and especially on Meyer's. His bureau had been the subject of a Senate inquiry three years before and needed nothing less than the black-marketing and discrimination characteristic of vaccine distribution in 1957.

To this group, enlarged by CDC staff, Dowdle reported his laboratory findings. The question at once became whether four human cases were the first appearance of incipient pandemic or a fluke of some kind, a limited transfer to a few humans of what remained an animal disease which would not thrive in people. All agreed that on the present evidence there was no means of knowing. Surveillance was the task at hand. Since their uncertainty was real, they agreed also that there should be no publicity until there were more data: why raise public concern about what might turn out an isolated incident? Some days later CDC scrapped this agreement on the plea that uninformed press leaks were imminent, and Sencer called a press conference for February 19. He must have hated the thought that an announcement might come from some place other than CDC. However that may be, the press conference got national attention.

In the *New York Times* Harold Schmeck reported, February 20:

The possibility was raised today that the virus that caused the greatest world epidemic of influenza in modern history—the pandemic of 1918–19—may have returned.

This story (on page 1) was headed:

U.S. Calls Flu Alert On Possible Return of Epidemic Virus

The 1918 reference was included in brief notices that night, on CBS and ABC news telecasts. NBC went them one better and showed 1918 still pictures of persons wearing masks. Lacking further information, the media did not follow up the story for a month. But 1918 left a trace in certain minds, some of them TV producers and reporters. From within CDC, we have encountered a good deal of retrospective criticism at press tendencies to "harp" on 1918 prematurely, with no evidence whatsoever about prospective virulence or even spread through 1976. These NBC pictures are cited along with the *New York Times* headline. But the reference was included in the CDC press briefing, and indeed without it, what was known about Fort Dix so far was scarcely news at all. What sense to a conference that did not bring it up?

Publicity had no effect upon the effort to establish what the Fort Dix outbreak meant. In Fort Dix itself, where the Army conducted its own investigation shielded from civilians, the Victoria strain proved dominant, at least for the time being. There were plenty of new influenza cases; none was caused by the swine virus. On the other hand, that virus was isolated from a fifth soldier who had been sick in early February, and blood tests confirmed eight more old cases of swine flu, none of them fatal. Moreover, a sampling of antibody levels among recruits suggested that as many as 500 had been infected by swine flu. This implied human transmission on a scale that could not reasonably be viewed lightly. Around Fort Dix, however, in the civilian population—which was Goldfield's territory for investigation—analysis of every case of flu reported, by a medical community on the alert, showed only Victoria. Elsewhere in New Jersey Goldfield's inquiries turned up no swine flu. The Army's inquiries turned up none at camps other than Fort Dix. The NIAID network of university researchers and the state epidemiologists in touch with CDC reported none untraceable to pigs. The World Health Organization, pressed by CDC, could learn of none abroad. One death, thirteen sick men and up to 500 recruits who evidently had caught and resisted the disease, all in one Army camp, were the only established instances of human-to-human swine flu found around the world as February turned into March, the last month of flu season in the Northern Hemisphere.

On March 10 the group that had met February 14 reassembled at CDC and under Sencer's chairmanship reviewed their findings with the Advisory Committee on Immunization Practices (ACIP). That committee was in form a set of outside experts appointed by the Surgeon General, independently advising CDC; in fact it was almost a part of CDC, nominated, chaired and staffed at Sencer's discretion. BoB deadlines now forced his pace. One ACIP function was to make vaccine recommendations for the next flu season available to manufacturers. The annual questions were: vaccine against what viruses, aimed at which population groups? For 1976 these questions had already been reviewed in a January ACIP meeting. The committee had recommended Victoria vaccine for the "high-risk groups" as then defined, some 40 million people over 65 in age or with certain chronic diseases. By March 10, the four active manufacturers had produced in bulk form about 20 million doses of Victoria vaccine for the civilian market. If Fort Dix meant a change or addition, now was the time to decide. Indeed, for a regulatory body like the BoB, responsible for setting standards and for quality control, March was already late. Vaccine is grown in eggs; a vaccine against swine flu would require new supplies replacing those just used for Victoria vaccine. Then immunization trials would be needed if there were a new vaccine; also extensive testing. And what about the vaccine now in bulk? Whatever surveillance had turned up by now would have to suffice for some sort of decision.

2

SENCER DECIDES

Sencer was an able, wily autocrat with a devoted staff. The CDC was wholly his. He knew everything about it, everybody in it, and took care to put his own imprint on policy. Swine flu was no exception.

He spent March 9 preparing for the ACIP meeting in informal get-togethers with his laboratory people and some other senior aides. Dowdle recalled when we interviewed him:

It was clear we could not say the virus would spread. But it was clear that there had been human-to-human spread at Fort Dix. It was also clear that there was not any immunity in the population to this virus, not if you were under 50 (or maybe 62). Usual "high-risk" categories did not apply. Most people were at risk, especially young adults. An epidemic spreading into a pandemic had to be anticipated *as a possibility*.

. . . Army recruits were a unique population group . . . maybe they would be the only ones affected. But the current disappearance of the virus did not prove that. Flu could do strange things. Six weeks was a short time. We had to report our fundamental belief that a pandemic was indeed a possibility.

This was the scientist speaking. What could not be disproved must be allowed for. Dowdle also recalls his frustration with the lack of data and his sadness at the thought of "changing all those lives," disrupting CDC by action on so little information. Influenza was a slippery phenomenon. Not much was known about pandemic spread. Aside from the three years of 1918, 1957, 1968, the past was mostly conjecture. And recorded spread in those years varied quite enough to buttress contradictory arguments about what now was happening. Since February, swine flu might have sunk back into pigs. Or was it spreading in humans subclinically, "seeding itself" to erupt explosively next flu season? Nothing quite like Fort Dix and the lack of spread beyond it had been seen before. One could guess but not know. And even among specialists, guesses diverged. Dowdle reportedly was cool to claims that a swine virus readily dominated by Victoria at Fort Dix would shortly arise and sweep around the world. In the circumstances he was not much afraid of subclinical spread. But others were: Kilbourne, for one, who would be with them the next day.

In the then hierarchy of virologists, as several tell us now, Dowdle was the Coming Man but Kilbourne an Old Great, while Sencer was a well-informed bystander. Of the few generally acknowledged "Greats" in Kilbourne's class, none was a current member of the ACIP and he himself would be there out of interest, not entitlement (he had just been appointed for a term not yet begun). His presence was to count. It counted more as others recall it than as he does.

Save for some epidemiologists, whose eyes shine even yet with remembered excitement, many CDC-ers were at least as cool as Dowdle on March 9. More precisely they remember being at once apprehensive and resigned. As one of those who sat through Sencer's staff sessions explained to us:

There was nothing in this for CDC except trouble. Here we were at the end of one flu season with time to try to do something before the next flu season. The obvious thing to do was immunize everybody. But if we tried to do that, guide it, help it along, we might have to interrupt a hell of a lot of work on other diseases . . . work here, and in the states, a lot of places.

Then if a pandemic came, lots of people—maybe millions— would be angry . . . because they couldn't get shots when they wanted. . . . Or they got sick of something else that they mistook for flu and thought our shots weren't working. Most people in this country (including half the doctors) call all kinds of things flu that aren't. As for "another 1918," I didn't expect that, but who could be sure? . . . It would wreck us.

Yet, on the other hand, if there weren't a pandemic we'd be charged with wasting public money . . . crying wolf . . . causing all that inconvenience for nothing . . . and not only the people who got shots . . . the people who administered the shots . . . our friends out in the states . . . what would they think of us? It was a no-win situation . . . we saw that . . . talked about it . . .

But institutional protection could not override the ethic of preventive medicine. Disease prevention was the professional commitment of them all, including those who cared for CDC the most. They felt themselves trapped. With a pandemic possible and time to do something about it, and lacking the time to disprove it, then *something* would have to be done. So ran the logic of what Sencer heard from his staff.

The next day, at the March 10 ACIP meeting, staff spelled out the situation (couched, of course, in Dowdle's terms, not those of institutional protection). It was an open meeting, though with minimal press attendance. After hours of discussion a consensus emerged:

First, the possibility of pandemic existed. None thought it negligible. Kilbourne thought it very likely. Most seem to have thought privately of likelihoods within a range from two to twenty percent; each was prepared to bet, however, with nobody but himself. These probabilities, after all, were based on personal judgment, not scientific fact. They voice them to us now; they did not voice them then.[4]

Second, while severity could not be estimated, one death in a dozen was worrisome. Besides, somewhere in everybody's mind lurked 1918. No one thought there literally could be a repetition; antibiotics would hold down the death rate from bacterial complications. Deaths aside, few thought the virus would be so severe. When last seen in the '20's it was mild. But nobody could bring himself to argue that such mildness was assured. It wasn't.

Third, traditional definition of high-risk groups did not apply. People under 50 had no natural protection, and young adults had suffered unusually high mortality in the 1918 pandemic. This argued for producing enough vaccine to inoculate them all before the next flu season. All meant all, or as many as possible, because one could not count on "herd" immunity to stifle epidemic spread. In influenza nothing on this scale had ever been attempted. But not since 1957 had the timing of discovery allowed for it. And then we did not have vaccines as safe or as effective as the ones developed since. Nor did we have the guns for swift injection. With a decision now, the manufacturers could buy their eggs and make the vaccine fast enough so that inoculations could begin in summer, when the chance of flu was slightest and the risk of panic least. Meanwhile, plans could be made for mass immunization.

Predisposition buttressed that consensus. It reflected the agendas several ACIP members drew from other aspects of their working lives. Kilbourne, for one, not only championed his theories, but was keen to make the country see the virtues of preventive medicine. Swine flu seemed to him a splendid opportunity. Others also saw the chance to demonstrate the value of public health practice. Dr. Reuel Stallones, Dean of the Public Health School at the University of Texas, recalled for us:

> This was an opportunity to try to pay something back to society for the good life I've had as a public health doctor. Society has done a lot for me—this is sheer do-goodism. It was also an opportunity to strike a blow for epidemiology in the interest of humanity. The rewards have gone overwhelmingly to molecular biology, which doesn't do much for humanity. Epidemiology ranks low in the hierarchy—in the pecking order, the rewards system. Yet it holds the key to reducing lots of human suffering.

Consensus thus supported might have dissolved over one issue which at this meeting was never joined: should one move automatically from ordering the vaccine and preparing for its use to using it? If so, what evidence about the spread of the disease would make one stop and stockpile it instead? If not, what evidence would make one move from stockpiling into mass immunization?

Dr. Russell Alexander of the Public Health School at the University of Washington was the principal proponent of a pause for further evidence. His concern was more medical than managerial. As he put it to us in retrospect:

My general view is that you should be conservative about putting foreign material into the human body. That's always true . . . especially when you are talking about 200 million bodies. The need should be estimated conservatively. If you don't need to give it, don't.

He also had a glimmering of one aspect of management, public understanding and acceptance. He told us:

If you have spread combined with high surveillance, then the surrounding communities will really go to work and the public will really cooperate each time flu is reported in a new place. If it hit Denver you could immunize Seattle, because everybody would move fast.

Alexander did not make a speech. He put in questions or made comments when he could. An unimpassioned man, he was so mild that other members we have seen recall but vaguely something about "stockpiling." He himself makes light of it. Known as a voice of caution in past meetings, he was easy to discount on this occasion. But Schmeck, the *New York Times* man, there as an observer, stressed to us:

Alexander seemed serious about stockpiling. He wanted to know "at what point do we stop going on with our preparations to immunize everybody and turn to stockpiling instead—what point in terms both of progress of our preparations and progress of the disease." He asked this seriously. It was not answered.

If so, the term "stockpiling" trivializes, even distorts, Alexander's question, which embraced not alone the issue of a waiting game but also the criteria for playing it. And failure to pursue them both, *especially* criteria, appears by hindsight sad, an opportunity lost. From this we draw a lesson for next time.

That they were not pursued in the ACIP meeting was Sencer's choice from the chair. It could not have escaped him that there was some nascent sentiment for separating manufacture from inoculation. Goldfield and a colleague, in particular, spoke for it from their vantage point, New Jersey, and were evidently bursting to elaborate, if asked. Sencer seems to have wanted none of that. The day before he had discussed stockpiling with his staff, and they had ended by dismissing it. Inoculation took two weeks to bring immunity. Infection brings on the disease within a few days. In two weeks flu could spread throughout a city. Add air travel and how prevent its spreading through the country unless everyone were immunized beforehand? Besides, there was the issue of response-time by state clinics, private doctors, volunteers, and citizens at large, the objects of it all. Even a short lag could be too long. "Jet-spread" and slow response combined to make a stockpile option moot. So staff had said.

Staff aside, Seal tells us he and Meyer talked with Sencer at some point. One of them, Seal no longer remembers which, observed for Sencer's benefit (one career executive to another):

Suppose there is a pandemic accompanied by deaths. Then it comes out: "They had the opportunity to save life; they made the vaccine, they put it in the refrigerator. . . ." That translates to "they did nothing." And worse, "they didn't even recommend an immunization campaign to the Secretary."

When it came to the ACIP, whose first task was to ponder manufacture, Sencer did not insist on drawing Alexander out, much less encourage Goldfield, and the March 10 meeting ended with the issue of what happened after manufacture blurred. The minutes of the meeting state: "It was, therefore, agreed that the production of vaccine must proceed and that a plan for vaccine administration be developed." Everybody present we have talked to says the same. That is as far as they got. Sencer recalled for us:

I went into the [ACIP] meeting with an open mind . . . We met all morning . . . By 2:00 or 2:30 a consensus had emerged . . . Stallones summed it up best: *First*, there was evidence of a new strain with man-to-man transmission. *Second*, always before when a new strain was found there was a subsequent pandemic. And *third*, for the first time, there was both the knowledge and the time to provide for mass immunization. So, he said, "if we believe in preventive medicine we have no choice." I asked the committee to sleep on it and let us phone them the next day to make sure they still felt the same way, which we did—and they did.

Sencer and his staff turned promptly to the practical effects of the consensus. This had never been considered ACIP business. Governmental consultation, legislation, budgeting, contracting and the like were not its charge. Implementation was Sencer's business. One ACIP member, who stayed over for a day and called upon some senior CDC officials, commented to us: "I found them all busy with planning and mostly unable to talk to me."

Sencer himself went to work with one aide and wrote a nine-page paper, known to all and sundry as his "action-memorandum." In the process, he recalls, he made up his own mind precisely what the Federal government should do. His paper was designed at once to say it and to sell it.

In form this memorandum was addressed to David Mathews, Secretary of HEW, from Dr. Theodore Cooper, the Assistant Secretary for Health, Sencer's boss. In fact it was to go on up from Mathews to the Office of Management and Budget (OMB), to the Domestic Council, to the White House, to President Ford, as *the* decision paper in the case. It was written for that purpose and it served so. Thus it has a special place in our decision-making story. It is worth reading in full and we include it in Appendix D.

Sencer began his memo with "Facts":

1. In February 1976 a new strain of influenza virus. . . .

2. The virus is antigenically related to the [one] implicated as the cause of the 1918–19 pandemic which killed 450,000 people—more than 400 of every 100,000 Americans.

3. The entire U.S. population under the age of 50 is probably susceptible to this new strain.

   . . .

   . . .

6. Severe epidemics, or pandemics, of influenza recur at approximately 10 year intervals. In 1968–69. . . .

7. A vaccine . . . can be developed before the next flu season; how-

ever, the production of large quantities would require extraordinary efforts by drug manufacturers.

CDC officials present and past, Sencer included, have complained to us about the overemphasis on 1918 at the Secretary's level and the White House. Here is where it began.

Sencer turned next to "Assumptions":

1. Although there has been only one outbreak . . . [there is] a strong possibility that this country will experience widespread . . . swine influenza in 1976–77. . . . major antigenic shift . . . population under 50 is almost universally susceptible . . . ingredients for a pandemic.
2. . . . Routine actions would have to be supplemented.
3. The situation is one of "go or no go" . . . there is barely enough time. . . . A decision must be made now.
4. There is no medical epidemiologic basis for excluding any part of the population [*i.e.*, everyone can catch it and don't count on "herd effect"] . . . it is assumed . . . socially and politically unacceptable to *plan* for less than 100 percent coverage. Therefore . . . any recommendations for action must be directed toward the goal of immunizing 213 million people in three months. . . .

Sencer still is seething about Ford and Cooper, who were soon to make exaggerated pledges of vaccine for everybody. But the drafters of their statements followed his lead.

The Sencer memorandum then got down to recommendations, offering four options of a sort common in government: three framed to be rejected by the reader, with the fourth the one desired by the writer. First was "do nothing," followed by a set of "pros" and "cons." Among the cons:

- The Administration can tolerate unnecessary health expenditures better than unnecessary death and illness . . .
- In all likelihood, Congress will act on its own initiative.

Second was "minimum response." This must have had some staff support in CDC. It proposed making vaccine for all, the government committed to buy part, whether used or not (for Federal beneficiaries in Medicare, Medicaid, Veterans Administration and Department of Defense), the other part available commercially, and everyone exhorted to get shots through normal channels. This was relatively cheap and also easy in administrative terms, nothing unprecedented about it (except numbers of doses and dollars). But among the "cons":

- There is little assurance that vaccine manufacturers will undertake the massive production effort . . . required. . . .
- . . . the poor, the near poor, and the aging usually get left out. . . .
- Probably only about half the population would get immunized.

Third was a "government program," Federal and state, without private physicians, and fourth was a "combined approach" which added a role for the private sector.

The fourth option was recommended. It envisaged Federal purchase of vaccine for everybody, production by the private manufacturers, field trials through NIAID, licensing by BoB, planning through the states, immunization through a mix of public-private services and surveillance through CDC. The estimated cost was $134 million: $100 million for vaccine, the rest for operations and surveillance or research. Administratively, as Sencer warned, this was a leap into the dark, "no precedents, nor mechanisms in place," and an heroic response to a dire possibility.

Sencer, in so recommending, may have played the hero in his own mind; if so, he was but the first who did. Mathews, Cooper and Ford, among others, would follow.

In retrospect, this action-memorandum reads as though it were deliberately designed to force a favorable response from a beset Administration that could not afford to turn it down and then to have it leak. The memorandum actually had that effect, but CDC associates doubt Sencer was deliberate. They think him "a physician with a conscience." They think he simply "meant to make the strongest case he could."

However that may be, Sencer rolled the felt need to do "something" into one decision: manufacture, planning, immunizing and surveillance all together, and tied the whole to Meyer's deadline for the manufacturers, those egg supplies. On their account the deadline was two weeks away, "go or no go."

3

COOPER ENDORSES

Sencer's paper was completed March 13 and he took it to Washington. On Monday morning, March 15, he met Secretary Mathews in an emergency session. This had been arranged by Cooper's deputy, Dr. James Dickson, who attended and brought Meyer. Cooper was in Cairo, keeping a long-planned engagement, but Dickson had his proxy; Cooper and Sencer had talked on the phone the week before (and Cooper had arranged to be reached, if wanted, through White House facilities).

Mathews had been in office only since the previous August. A gracious man and graceful, he had left the Presidency of the University of Alabama, where he had deep roots (and to which he would return), for a Department where he was almost unknown. Seven months had scarcely changed that; he remained but a name to most of Cooper's people. Moreover, they were unaware that by his own account to us he had brought with him a deep feeling for preventive medicine. He thinks that he and they were philosophically in tune. From what they tell us, most of them would find the thought surprising.

Before seeing Sencer, the Secretary held his daily staff meeting. Dickson filled in for Cooper. Mathews' custom was to go around the circle of his operating chiefs and principal staff officers. When Dickson's turn came he described the swine flu problem much as Sencer's paper had done: "strong possibility." The meeting dissolved then and there in stories of 1918. As one participant explained to us, "We understood it might not happen . . . but lots of us had tales to tell about what it might be like if it did. . . ."

The meeting with Sencer followed. Sencer pushed Mathews hard. He did not rely on his paper (who does?), he enlarged upon it. He had been bracing for this meeting and apparently was worried about it. In PHS, Mathews was often called "the phantom," all too readily dismissed as uninformed, uninterested and, worse, uninfluential at such crucial places as the OMB. Sencer was in budgetary trouble and he had been for some years. President Nixon's New Federalists—still more James Lynn, Ford's Budget Director—liked discretionary funds for states and maximum reliance upon private medicine. CDC believed in limiting discretion to assure results. Also, it drew sustenance from categorical grants and wanted more of them. Under the Republicans, both OMB and planning staffs at PHS had sought to hold back new departures and to trim the old. Revenue-sharing with the states plus Medicare and Medicaid, *not* project grants through CDC, had seemed to them the way to go.

Sencer's memorandum is expressive of his worries:

Given this situation can we afford the administrative and programmatic inflexibility that would result from normal considerations about duplicative costs, third party reimbursements and Federal-State or public-private relationships and responsibilities? The magnitude of the challenge suggests that the Department must either be willing to take extraordinary steps or be willing to accept an approach to the problem that cannot succeed.

From what others tell us, Sencer pressed Mathews harder than he need have done. He evidently underestimated either the sheer force of his own message unadorned, or Mathews, or perhaps both. Dickson remembers:

I presented the issue to Mathews. . . . He said to me, "What's the probability?" I said, "Unknown." From the look on Mathews' face when I said that, you could take it for granted that this decision was going to be made.

Mathews bears him out, commenting to us:

The moment I heard Sencer and Dickson, I *knew* the "political system" would *have* to offer some response. No way out, unless they were far out from the center of scientific consensus (a small band of people in influenza). They weren't—although some of those people waffled later. So it was inevitable. . . .

As for the *possibility* of another 1918 . . . one had to assume the *probability* greater than zero. If they say "unknown" that's the least they can mean. Well, that's enough for action if you know in time. You can't face the electorate later, if it eventuates, and say well, the probability was so low we decided not to try, just two or five percent, you know, so why spend the money. The "political system" should, perhaps, but *won't* react that way. . . . So again, it's inevitable.

Moreover, Mathews recalls favoring the substance, risk aside. Sencer, in his view, would have been wrong had he conceived Administration preferences for state and private medicine as tantamount to lack of faith in immunization programs. These Mathews remembers liking. He recalls thinking the addition of a flu program desirable even had the risk seemed far away.

Dickson recalls something more in Mathews' reaction:

. . . politically impossible to say no, but more, it's what "unknown" conveyed to [Mathews] about the risk in human terms . . . lives. . . . It didn't seem to him remote at all.

Meyer, listening, watching, took relatively little part until late. This was not shyness, just prudence. He recalls some discomfort at Sencer's "hard sell" but never having met Mathews before, he was unsure of the ground rules. As he put it to us:

I felt uncomfortable about the firmness, absoluteness with which Sencer put the issue and the decision to the Secretary. Yet being a stranger to the Secretary I was hesitant about having rows with Sencer over tone.

Meyer remembers making two main points: The first was that with the uncertainty of a pandemic and likely reactions if none appeared, "everybody should be brought into the act. . . ." The second, in response to Mathews' inquiry, concerned safe manufacture of enough vaccine up to the proper standard: "a hell of a job" but it could be done.

The meeting ended on that note.

Then, or sometime after, Mathews heard of a new book, just out, coincidentally, *Epidemic and Peace, 1918*, by Alfred Crosby. Mathews promptly ordered copies and sent them to associates in HEW, the Budget and the White House. He also gave one to Ford.

Late in the morning of March 15, Mathews wrote a note to Lynn, the Director of the Budget:

> There is evidence there will be a major flu epidemic this coming fall. The indication is that we will see a return of the 1918 flu virus that is the most virulent form of flu. In 1918 a half million people died. The projections are that this virus will kill one million Americans in 1976.
>
> To have adequate protection, industry would have to be advised now in order to have time to prepare the some 200 million doses of vaccine required for mass inoculation. The decision will have to be made in the next week or so. We will have a recommendation on this matter since a supplemental appropriation will be required.

Note the escalation since the ACIP meeting five days earlier. There, except for the expectant Kilbourne, members tell us they had in their heads such likelihoods of epidemic spread as two or 20 percent, which translate into odds of 49:1 or 4:1 *against*. Nobody there explicitly equated spread with the severity of 1918. Kilbourne expected something relatively mild. Others may have thought the single figure in their minds applied quite separately to spread and to severity. A 2-percent chance of a 2-percent chance is exceedingly long odds. Sencer's memorandum then converts these (mostly unacknowledged) odds into "strong possibility" of a pandemic "antigenically related" to 1918: writing about spread he hints at severity, but never anywhere commits himself. Now Mathews, after their Monday meeting, equates spread with severity, converts the possible into the certain, "will," and with a doubled population he projects twice the casualties of fifty years ago. Had Sencer's case so moved him? Had he simply not thought it through? Or was he impressing his addressee, the Budget Director? Perhaps some of each.

Lynn already had heard something of this. So had his deputy, Paul O'Neill, the bright young man of OMB in Lyndon Johnson's time (beginning as a health programs examiner) who since had had a meteoric rise. O'Neill consulted with his colleague in the White House "deputies club," James Cavanaugh, soon to become deputy to Richard Cheney, the chief of staff.

Cavanaugh was then still Deputy Director of the Domestic Council, handling "operations" (which meant processing the day-to-day particulars). He had formerly been the health man on the Council's staff and liked to keep his hand in. His successor, Spencer Johnson, was brand new. A notable survivor, Cavanaugh had come to HEW in John Gardner's time, continued as a staffer under Robert Finch, briefly been Acting Assistant Secretary for Health and then been "loaned" by Elliot Richardson to John Ehrlichman when the Domestic Council was first formed. There, remarkably, Cavanaugh remained and even flourished under Ford, while the Council's Director, James Cannon, Vice President Rockefeller's choice, dealt with policy issues in the longer run.

Cavanaugh already had the ball, more or less, Cooper having warned him before leaving town. Dickson sent the Sencer memorandum over and Cavanaugh checked it out. The man with whom he chose to check was an old boss, Dr. Charles Edwards, Cooper's predecessor, now out of government. Edwards, hearing Cavanaugh's account, said, as the latter tells us, that from what he'd heard he'd go with Sencer, "the only possible course." Cooper, returning March 21, emphatically agreed. For Cavanaugh this sufficed. Johnson had inherited a duty to spy out the second and third echelons in HEW, although his acquaintance barely extended to Rockville, much less Atlanta. Cavanaugh saw no need to use him.

O'Neill, meanwhile, who had the final action since new money was involved, heard grumbling from his health examiners. Victor Zafra, the division chief, had read the *New York Times* of February 20 and had been waiting since for CDC to come in crying doom. He and his assistants deeply suspected a cooked-up job. Their relations with technicians inside PHS, however, were too strained or distant to give them a grip on anything like Alexander's worry (not, at least, in the short time available). So they wrapped their suspicions, instead, in classic budgetary guise, questioning the estimates. To quote from their internal memorandum:

PHS did not consider the possibility of reprogramming funds . . . we are not convinced that the $134 million estimate is a hard figure. . . . We think the figure could be trimmed down considerably using alternative assumptions and divisions of responsibility among the Federal and State governments and the private sector.

Tactically this could not help but fail by light of Sencer's urgency. O'Neill and Lynn saw that at once and although they too were suspicious—having Sencer in their sights—forbore to press the point. They did ask whether a new authorization was required to support appropriations; the examiners, along with Cooper's aides, said no (perhaps too flat an answer but accepted). Objections become harder still if nothing is needed but money.

Cavanaugh recalls pursuing other subjects, among them the idea of going for vaccine production right away while holding off a bit on choosing among options for its distribution. He spoke with "somebody at HEW" and was told no: "jet spread." He did not argue. The thought occurred to others besides him. At some point in the week before decision, as he told us:

There was a discussion between the President and the Vice President, after some meeting or other, in which Rockefeller said maybe one should go over to the Pentagon and get hold of a logistics officer and figure out how to do inoculations [throughout the country] in two to four weeks, thus beating "jet spread." Those were the time limits we'd been given and we also had been told they were too *tight* for manageable mass-immunization. Rockefeller's attitude was "HEW just doesn't know how, but I'll bet the military do." The thought wasn't followed up.

In Ford's Administration, few of Rockefeller's were.

If Cavanaugh was serious about distinguishing immunization from production he did not press the point. The others around Ford whom we have seen heard nothing of it, did not think of it themselves and doubt they would have liked it had they thought about it. O'Neill remarked to us:

As HEW presented the issue the time factor was key, not only to production—egg supplies—but to protection of the population before winter. Everybody by November. That's what Sencer was saying. So why decide twice? Commit now and be done with it. There isn't time at the White House to create *extra* decisions for the man to make. He's got plenty as it is.

Besides, Sencer was ready to press *his* case. If we held off on part of it how would the President look: Pennypincher? Trading lives for bucks? Indecisive? Can't make up his mind?

Besides, the case was not now simply Sencer's. Cooper, returning, had made it his own. And Cooper was trusted in quarters where Sencer was suspect ("manipulative"), not least in the Domestic Council and the White House. Cooper very often, as his aides report, mistrusted Sencer too. Sencer was 800 miles away and played his own game and had wherewithal to do it. This is a formula to drive a strong Assistant Secretary to distraction. Cooper certainly had strength and we gather was often distracted. A mercurial man, he was sometimes very angry. Yet here he showed himself an instant convert to Sencer's cause.

How did it come about that those two were together on this matter at this moment? The question is intriguing and important; the answer is elusive; we may not have fathomed its depths. But what we find is clear. First, Cooper respected Sencer's professional judgment, all the more so on an issue outside his own specialty (he was trained as a cardiac surgeon). Second, Cooper had a personal agenda into which Sencer's proposals fit. As leader and trustee of Federal services for health (which is, we think, how Cooper saw himself) he had been seeking ways to raise the consciousness of private citizens—of voluntary agencies, of parents, of physicians—to *prevention* of diseases through immunization and other means. Now there were vaccines for many infectious diseases; later, perhaps, for neurological disorders, conceivably even cancers. An associate commented to us:

Cooper had a strong sense of the importance of volunteer organizations and our dependence on them and the need to change and perfect them for the tasks ahead. . . . He wanted to move immediately onto a new footing, steadily supported by the voluntary groups and by parents all across the country—not subject to unpredictable shifts of government priorities. He was keen to increase comprehension of preventive medicine and support for it out there in the private sector where it could be shielded from those governmental ups and downs . . . those Nixon economy drives. . . .

Third, Cooper's father, a physician, had told him ghastly tales about 1918. He and Dickson, who also had a father with grim stories on the subject, traded recollections back and forth. The "worst case" possibility was vivid in the mind of the Assistant Secretary for Health.

Dickson mentioned to us:

Cooper really feared 1918. Something happened in Hershey, Pennsylvania, that stuck in Cooper's mind. They'd had to call out the troops to bury people *en masse*—they died so fast.

So Cooper, from the time Sencer first talked to him in February, was prepared to take an activist approach, provided it had backing from the "scientific community," that is to say from the relevant experts. He wanted to be sure that anything from CDC was first reviewed by the ACIP, and had support from NIAID, BoB and *their* advisers. Not leaving anything to others, Cooper himself talked to Dr. Albert Sabin. The latter's live vaccine for polio (superseding in this country Dr. Jonas Salk's killed-virus vaccine) had been used in the last nationwide mass immunization, 100 million in two seasons, "half the number in twice the time" that Sencer was now seeking. Sabin was encouraging, as Cooper knew when Sencer phoned him to report affirmatively on the ACIP meeting. So Cooper left for Cairo confident he could support what Sencer came up with. When he returned he did.

Meanwhile, his colleagues had gone to the President.

4

FORD ANNOUNCES

President Ford first heard of HEW's request for supplemental funds and all these entailed the afternoon of Monday, March 15, when Lynn, O'Neill and Cavanaugh met with him on another project. Three days later Ford heard somewhat more from Mathews and agreed to have a full review the following week.

It was a busy time for all concerned, not least for Ford. Swine flu was by no means the biggest item on his agenda. Among other things, presidential primaries were under way. Ford narrowly defeated Ronald Reagan in New Hampshire and had picked up strength in the next four primaries, especially the March 9 battle in Florida, where Reagan had hoped for an upset. On the same day, Ford had improved his position by telling Cheney to get rid of their lackluster campaign manager, Bo Callaway. But Ford's confidence was to be shaken by Reagan's surprise victory in North Carolina on Tuesday, March 23.

The day before the North Carolina primary, Lynn and O'Neill with Mathews, Cooper, Cheney, Cannon, Cavanaugh and Johnson met the President to review HEW's recommendation. From Lynn he got a packet in advance, including as was customary a summary paper with "talking points," questions for Mathews and Cooper. This was backed by Sencer's action-memorandum. In between was an OMB attachment labeled "Uncertainties Surrounding a Federal Mass Swine Influenza Immunization Program." Into this Lynn's aides had poured the hardest questions they could think of (or extract from other sources) on short notice. It was not a very arresting list. For what it's worth we include it in Appendix D. Cooper made short work of it. Someone on Mathews' staff or Cooper's had prepared a swine flu flip chart. Ford made short work of that. As one of his auditors says, he "blew up . . . waved it away," sensibly preferring discussion.

By all accounts the discussion ranged widely, covering at once the arguments for action, and a long list of drawbacks: The pandemic might not come and then the President would seem a spendthrift and alarmist, or a bumbler. If it came, the states and private sector might be overwhelmed, or seem so— "however well they did, it wouldn't be enough"—and he'd be blamed, again a bumbler. Or vaccine might not be ready soon enough. Uncertainty about the egg supply meant, ultimately, roosters. The Secretary of Agriculture had been reassuring: "The roosters of America are ready to do their duty. . . ." Still, yield per egg of vaccine might be less than was wanted. And so forth. As one participant recalls:

I told the President that this was a no-win position politically. There was no good to come of it as far as the election was concerned . . . if there were no pandemic a lot of people would have sore arms in October. If there were a pandemic, no matter how much we'd done it wouldn't be enough and he'd be roundly criticized.

Others tell us they said much the same, but one of them remembers thinking (and, he hopes, saying):

There is no way to go back on Sencer's memo. If we tried to do that, it would leak. That memo's a gun to our head.

Among the things Ford was *not* warned about were six: trouble with serious side effects, with children's dosages, with liability insurance, with expert opinion, with PHS public relations, and with his own credibility. On the contrary, the vaccine was presumed both safe and efficacious; insurance was not known to be a problem; experts were pronounced on board; Cooper and Sencer could cope with the press. And while the venture's cost to Ford in public terms was aired, nobody raised the opposite, the burden to the program of *his* sponsorship amidst a problematic fight for the Republican nomination.

These six are the drawbacks that in fact would give the effort the bad name it has today among attentive publics. Some of them may not have been foreseeable, as most of Ford's aides tell us now. For what it may be worth, we tend to disagree. At least it can be said that signs of each were somewhere to be seen had staffers penetrated far enough. But with agendas of their own, or sitting on the sidelines, or beset by other work, they didn't.

Hearing what he heard, Ford saw the issue simply. Politics had no part in it. As he recalled when we saw him:

I think you ought to gamble on the side of caution. I would always rather be ahead of the curve than behind it. I had a lot of confidence in Ted Cooper and Dave Mathews. They had kept me informed from the time this was discovered. Now Ted Cooper was advocating an early start on immunization, as fast as we could go, especially in children and old people. So that was what we ought to do, unless there were some major technical objection.

This agrees with what others remember. Some may have been pleased that what was right to do was also politic, one-upping Reagan: Here would be the *President*, decisive for the public good. Others, though, were worried by the public risks Ford ran in longer terms. Mathews recalled for us:

I told him that I knew it was a no-win situation for him, and that it wasn't necessary for him to make the announcement—I said I would do it if he wished me to.

Two of Ford's aides had talked of this, but Mathews was a weak reed in their eyes and anyway, "we thought he'd punted." Besides, the President seemed quite content, some even thought him eager, to announce a swine flu program as his own and urge public support of it. He evidently thought then, and still does, that this was his plain duty: "If you want to get 216 million people immunized this requires the imprimatur of the White House." Like Mathews, Cooper and Sencer, Ford may also have had a refreshing sense of doing a direct, uncomplicated, decently heroic deed.

So Mathews' offer was not pursued. Cooper tells us that *he* would have been glad, even then, to make the announcement himself. The same can be said of Sencer, who wishes they had simply let him walk the supplemental up to the House Appropriations Committee and announce it there. Nothing like that was suggested to Ford by Cooper or anyone else.

The meeting of March 22 did not end with a final decision. Instead, the President decided to postpone decision until he had heard the views of experts in the field outside the government, the scientific community personified. O'Neill, who pressed the point, remembered in our interview:

I really felt strongly that the President should meet a representative group of "scientists" in advance. In private conversations we had found no discernible dissent. . . . The President, of necessity, had to rely very heavily on their scientific judgment. . . . I thought they ought to be willing to commit themselves publicly.

Ford himself seems to have seen still more in this, not only shoring up his credibility but genuinely reaching for advice. Like Mathews before him he had been told that a swine flu pandemic, shades of 1918, was "possible," but that the probability remained "unknown." (Cooper refused to put any numbers on it, although once he offered "one to 99.") If those words meant what Ford took them to mean, justifying an unprecedented Federal action, he wanted to be sure the experts felt the same, or know if some did not, and why, and wanted to hear it from them at first hand. Lacking a science adviser (the post was in abeyance then), he asked, as he recalls, that the "best" scientists (along with experts on such things as manufacturing) be brought together with him two days hence. Others recall his asking for "a full spectrum" of scientific views. Either way, he ended this first meeting on that note.

Cavanaugh undertook to assemble the required experts in

consultation with Cooper, who consulted in turn with Sencer and Meyer, among others. The list of expert invitees as they contrived it included Kilbourne, Stallones, Dr. Frederick Davenport (a noted virologist), Maurice Hilleman (the respected head of Merck virology labs), and as a crowning touch *both* Salk and Sabin. These two were outside the ACIP circle—which to Cavanaugh assured a spectrum—and were inveterate opponents, personally and professionally. To Cavanaugh this meant that if there were clay feet on Sencer's program, Salk would be the man to find them (Sabin having indicated his support). If they agreed, despite their enmity, this should assure the President the "best support available." They, at any rate, were by far the best *known* to press and public.

Alexander was not on the list. Cavanaugh did not know him. The others, juggling numbers, did not propose him.

No members of Congress were on the list either. Several were due to be informed by phone, but no one proposed to have them in the meeting. The Senate subcommittee chairman most interested, Edward Kennedy, had been lambasting Ford for a retreat on health insurance. No one proposed Kennedy; if not him, nobody. Besides, in retrospect at least, the aides with whom we've spoken are convinced it would have seemed either "political" or "weak" for Ford to have brought in the opposition to share *his* decision.

On March 24, at 3:30 P.M., Ford met his scientists and some others from the states, the AMA and so forth, in the Cabinet Room. He was accompanied by a full complement of aides and HEW officials. Sencer opened with a briefing. The President then turned to Salk, who strongly urged mass immunization. In back rows aides sighed with relief. Salk recalled for us:

When the President asked for comment I made the points that influenza was indeed an important disease, and that the program was an opportunity to educate the public and to justify further research. . . . I don't think I then said but I certainly thought of it as a great opportunity to fill part of the "immunity gap" [between antigens in our environment and populations without antibodies]. We should close the gap whenever we can. Here was a chance. . . . That's what I saw in the program, so of course I supported it.

Sabin followed Salk, then Hilleman, and then the President asked others to chime in. He went around the table seeking views as if he really wanted them, which indeed he did. His respondents saw that and it gratified them but it also puzzled them. Summoned to the White House on short notice, many for the first time, ushered into a large, formal meeting, watching Ford call first on one and then another, most of those we've interviewed took it to be "programmed," a "stage set" and they "players" . . . "the decision taken" . . . "we were used."

Indeed it had been programmed, oddly enough twice. Stallones recalled for us a call from Sencer, the night before, to tell him when to speak and what the President would ask. The "talking points" Ford got from Johnson were, however, different in detail. Sencer evidently had to vie for programming with the Domestic Council.

At some point in the meeting, Ford asked for a show of hands on whether to proceed. All hands went up. He then asked whether there were any dissents or objections, on the other side. A long silence ensued. One of the experts present tells us now:

> Later, I regretted not having spoken up and said, "Mr. President, this may not be proper for me to say, but I believe we should not go ahead with immunization until we are sure this is a real threat."

However that may be, it wasn't said.

Earnestly in his mind, though *pro forma* to his listeners, the President then observed that he would be glad to talk to anyone who had doubts for his ear alone. He would suspend the meeting and would wait a few moments in the Oval Office. So he did.

While waiting, Ford reviewed with Cavanaugh and others the announcement he would make and when to make it. If done at once, it could but strengthen the impression of a "programmed" meeting (so, in fact, it did). But if delayed, the television news that night and then the morning papers might be filled with separate interviews from leaky scientists. One of Ford's advisers said to us in retrospect:

> . . . the net result might be a speculative spate of news stories and editorials which either scared people or presented them with the

impression of an imminent national emergency or made it look as though the President couldn't make up his mind.

Or the press might charge him with deliberate stalling to create a media event. And Ford himself, remembering the moment, added in his talk with us: "If you've got unanimity, you'd better *go* with it. . . ."

So he went. He stopped by the Cabinet Room, collared both Sabin and Salk, waved good-bye to the others, and continued to the Press Room, over the old swimming pool, with its facilities for instant briefing. Then and there with Salk and Sabin flanking him, he announced his decision:

I have been advised that there is a very real possibility that unless we take effective counteractions, there could be an epidemic of this dangerous disease next fall and winter here in the United States.

Let me state clearly at this time: no one knows exactly how serious this threat could be. Nevertheless, we cannot afford to take a chance with the health of our nation. Accordingly, I am today announcing the following actions.

. . . I am asking the Congress to appropriate $135 million, prior to their April recess, for the production of sufficient vaccine to inoculate every man, woman, and child in the United States.

Sabin spoke up also. Mathews and Cooper then took questions.

The reporters were relatively well-prepared. To Cavanaugh's chagrin, a "Fact Sheet" for the briefing had arrived while Ford was still consulting in the Cabinet Room. Simultaneously, a group of White House aides had called the subcommittee chairmen and some others on the Hill to give them advance warning. Word of this began to trickle back. And two days earlier, John Cochran of NBC News had scooped his confreres with a story on the Monday meeting. They had been boning up on swine flu since.

Cochran, who had Alabama ties, got wind on Sunday night that Mathews had a White House meeting the next day, and pulled its purpose out of sources in the Secretary's Office. He then got it confirmed, still more reluctantly, from White House aides who feared it would be played "sensationally" in a way to preempt Ford or scare the public. When NBC ran a straightforward, circumspect account instead, they were relieved.

Cochran and Robert Pierpoint of CBS, among others, thereupon proceeded to the question they, as White House correspondents, had to ask: was this political? Those two went about seeking answers differently. In reportorial terms, one way seems as good as the other. Cochran ranged across the list of Ford's political advisers, covering them thoroughly, we believe, from top to bottom without finding an enthusiast among them. This made a lasting impression. He was ready, thereafter, to assume the politicians felt compelled to do the bidding of the experts. Pierpoint, hearing that his bureau in Atlanta had some input, called and got an earful. A local CBS man had been following the story. With his interest heightened by the coverage on NBC he had called sources inside CDC, professional sources, experts, and been told on *deep* background that, given present evidence, nationwide immunization was unjustified, "a crazy program," or words to that effect. Sencer's advocacy they attributed to obscure pressure on him from above, to some "political" motive he, for reasons unknown, could not resist. Doctors often use the term "political" for anything that isn't "scientific." To the CBS reporters, and especially to Pierpoint, it could have only one meaning in this case. He was so exercised that he persuaded his superiors to put his findings in the same story as Ford's announcement of March 24. The Cronkite show that night had Pierpoint saying:

Some experts seriously question whether it is logistically possible to inoculate two hundred million Americans by next fall. But beyond that, some doctors and public health officials have told CBS News that they believe that such a massive program is premature and unwise, that there is not enough proof of the need for it, and it won't prevent more common types of flu. But because President Ford and others are endorsing the program, those who oppose it privately are afraid to say so in public.

A day later all three networks aired dissent from open sources, mainly Dr. Sidney Wolfe, a frequent critic of the public health establishment. But the critics Pierpoint mentioned were the ones who left a mark at CBS. For him, for his bureau chief in Washington and for at least some of the Cronkite show's producers, Ford's program was forever suspect: dubious in expert eyes, hence probably political. As one of them put it to us:

It was a rotten program, rotten to the core. We thought it was politically inspired . . . it certainly was awful in technical terms . . . unwarranted . . . unnecessary. That impression came straight from CDC. We didn't get onto Wolfe until later.

It might be that the President himself had been imposed upon. Pierpoint liked Cavanaugh and thought him a good citizen. As both remember, Pierpoint called to tell him (without revealing sources) that there was dissenting medical opinion *in* the government. Cavanaugh was startled, having heard none, nor had Cooper, nor had Mathews. Sencer had reported unanimity from the ACIP, polled on the phone, and so had Meyer from polling a panel of his own. Sencer's polling may have been a bit contrived; one member told us he remembers hearing that an all-out program was required for congressional approval, another that the White House was insisting on immunization. Cavanaugh knew nothing of such details. Besides, there was no going back; the thing was done.

5

ORGANIZING

Congress responded promptly to the President's call for funds. An appropriation in precisely the amount requested was tacked onto a pending supplemental bill by an accommodating Senate Appropriations Committee. It was voted by the Senate April 9, by the House April 12, and signed into law April 15. The substantive health subcommittees, especially in the House, wanted and saw need for authorizing legislation, which the House indeed passed, but the Senate acted on the appropriation only. Chairman Paul G. Rogers of the House Health Subcommittee and Chairman Edward M. Kennedy, his Senate counterpart, both held hearings on the substance of the swine flu threat. So did the chairmen of the relevant House and Senate subcommittees on appropriations. Sencer testified at all hearings, but Cooper, who also testified on each occasion, was the star witness, particularly with the substantive committees. He had credibility at both ends of the Avenue, no mean feat in 1976. He was taken quite as seriously by Kennedy and Rogers as by Cavanaugh and Ford. And what he told them was what Ford had told the country:

By reviewing the epidemiology and natural history of this process, we do feel that a strong possibility exists that in the next flu season . . . there is a good likelihood that there will be influenza caused by this particular agent. . . .

The strain is related to the swine influenza virus which has been implicated as the cause of the 1918–19 pandemic. This pandemic caused approximately one-half million deaths in the United States alone.

I would not be happy with a 70–80 percent response. . . . I would like to make sure that we reach 95 percent . . . but our target population is a large one. My aspiration is for no less than 95 percent.

In retrospect Cooper told us wryly: "One lesson is 'watch your mouth.'" His overstatement of achievable objectives ran with Ford's: 95 percent amounted to about 200 million people. This pained some of the specialists at CDC who looked at the acceptance rates on past immunizations, together with exemptions for allergic persons, infants, and the very ill, and never dreamed of trying to inoculate more than 150 million.[5] They said to themselves "politics" and shrugged it off. The legislators, on the other hand, took Cooper's word as "science" and they gave him what he asked. He himself thinks now that he should have stopped first to figure out precisely what result would *satisfy* him, then distinguished that from any wider aims. He takes this as a lesson for next time.

In anticipation of the money, there was a short struggle over its administration. As early as March 13, Sencer at CDC had called on the director of his Bureau of State Services, Dr. Donald Millar, to head a planning task force. On April 2, at a meeting with state health officials, Sencer introduced Millar as "manager" of the prospective "National Influenza Immunization Program." Yet a week later in Washington, with funds at hand, Cooper by press release conferred the same title on Dr. Delano Meriwether of the PHS staff.

The coincidence of titles infuriated Sencer, but he seems not to have been the target of the tactic. This, rather, was the Secretary, who as Cooper's aides recall showed an uncharacteristic (and to them a quite unrealistic) interest in the running of the swine flu program.

Mathews had been energized by Ford, who looked to him for action. Besides, the swine flu program seemed to him a proper task, unlike so much of what his department did. Much of HEW left him cold. He was a believer in the states and a university administrator. Also, he considered it the Secretary's role to be a gap-filler, a "defensive secondary," becoming active only when the roles of none of his subordinates were wide enough. Sencer covered only CDC while Cooper added NIAID and BoB, but not the General Counsel (OGC) or others.

As we piece it together from associates (Mathews himself has less precise recollections), in the first days after March 15 he encouraged Jack Young, HEW's comptroller, to help Dickson design a swine flu organization. This would function under a departmentwide committee meeting daily. Young was a NASA alumnus from the moon-shot days. He and Dickson may have suspected what was coming at them operationally. Young's organization chart had certain interesting features, among them a place for program review, another for media relations. But Cooper would have none of it. No new organization could be built in time, "Flu season would have come and gone." In this he had concurrence from a crucial ally, with whom on other subjects he had often tangled horns, the Assistant Secretary for Planning and Evaluation, William Morrill, known in PHS as the Department's "other strong man." Cooper also thought—and Morrill seems to have agreed—that a committee under Mathews' wing would be a hopeless case and a committee meeting daily an abomination. Feeling responsible, welcoming the challenge, Cooper saw himself in charge, at least as much attracted to the task as Mathews and better equipped to do it.

Cooper's problem then was to keep Mathews at bay. Dickson was loyal and shut up. Young had no personal stake. Morrill was accommodating. The departmental committee, which soon started to meet weekly, then less frequently, never worked as Mathews wanted. And Meriwether was announced as Program Manager. A program with a manager is, *ipso facto*, organized.

Mathews went along, never having thought to run the thing alone, or without Cooper, and in no shape to hold out against him. As one of Mathews' aides told us:

Coming in only a year before the Republican Convention, that late in the Administration, we had no troops with which to challenge the "health division." To have had any chance of doing that, we'd have had to strip the University of Alabama clean of *all* Mathews' cadre of experienced assistants. We couldn't do that!

For his part, Sencer had been quite prepared to do it all through CDC, with NIAID and BoB and anybody else coordinated by Millar or by himself for working purposes. He would gladly have left it as Cooper's task—and Mathews' for that matter—to back them up. "The trouble was," Sencer commented to us, "that Cooper was looking for work; he had nothing much else to do. . . . That Administration had stifled all initiatives. The place was at a dead stop." In Cooper's perspective the trouble, of course, was different. It lay in Sencer's limited authority, distance from Washington, and personal style. How could he coordinate two other, equal agencies? How keep the White House happy, or the Washington press corps? And how carefully would he attend to the concerns of the Assistant Secretary? Sencer was not noted for that.

So Cooper sought to limit CDC to tasks he recognized it could do better than other existing agencies: encourage planning by the states, set standards and allot administrative funds to them, purchase the vaccine for them, and conduct surveillance. He was eager to include private physicians, also voluntary agencies—this indeed was one of his main interests in the program—but he had to hope state health departments would make these arrangements with encouragement enough from CDC. Perhaps this was expecting water to run uphill; time-pressures, in his view, left him no choice.

As for liaison with the vaccine manufacturers, field trials and testing, or related research, NIAID would do its job; so would BoB, coordinated as need be with CDC and states in usual informal ways or on appeal to Cooper. Meriwether would be his staff man for that; also for congressional, White House and press relations. Meriwether was a dedicated public health professional, loyal to his boss, an upright, high-achieving black with the stamina of an Olympic track star. What got beyond him Cooper would take on himself.

This arrangement cut out hordes of planners in the PHS but Cooper liked to travel light. Besides, in his opinion, as he told us, "nobody there knew anything about it." The arrangement also kept at arm's length PHS's Public Information staff, known then as one of the Department's best. No one recalls why they were so little used, except that Meriwether was a one-man band, and was meant to be.

Cooper, in the words of a collaborator, "trusted his capacity to doctor his way through." He sought to duck committees, stay lean, work fast and keep control. The scheme had two major flaws. The Department's General Counsel worked for Mathews, not for Cooper, a matter of small moment in April. (July would be another story when legal issues moved center stage.) And the media worked for themselves, on ground rules no M.D. in ·PHS seems to have fully understood.

There was, besides, Sencer's irritation with the Meriwether title, which he never ceased to think a clumsy and intrusive complication of Millar's essential role. But since the states looked to Millar in any case, while Washington press mostly went to Meriwether, and nobody there mistook him long for boss instead of staffer, it is hard to see what harm was caused except to Sencer's feelings. He, indeed, sanctioned the loan of a key man in Millar's bureau to be Meriwether's general-purpose aide. From July this kept lines open through the whole of the hard times ahead.

Inside CDC there was no jockeying at all, or rather what there was Sencer suppressed. Millar and his associates were soon working on three main lines:

First, they put together a PERT system, a way of charting all relations among things to be done in order to identify and treat impending bottlenecks. Although prepared by amateurs, it was pursued with gusto and may actually have helped. It also offered visual demonstration that the CDC could do a piece of project management as stylishly as NASA or the Navy. (Millar's master chart was on display for visitors—and still is.)

Second, they expanded and computerized the CDC's surveillance system. Dr. Michael Hattwick, who had urged this course for years, was put in charge with funds for staff and the computer of his dreams. He recruited a young statistician right out of graduate school and enticed young epidemiologists from other duties. Together they developed disease indicators matched imaginatively with reporting sources. The upshot was a center, manned around the clock, with all the verve and the devotion of a war room on alert. The public health community had never had anything like it, and the men who manned it trained hard for the task of tracking (beating) swine flu if (when) it should come. They wanted to be first to spot new outbreaks and they wanted to be sure about the timing, scale and consequences of mass immunization.

Hattwick himself was eager to track neurological complications. He recalls that he expected side effects upon the nervous system of some vaccinees—Guillain-Barré syndrome was one of three likely prospects—but he had no notion on what scale. As he put it to us: "We knew there would be some neurological complications. What we didn't know was just how frequently they would occur." No one then expected a high frequency and no one then explored the policy implications of low frequency, although each case could matter in the absence of pandemic. Policy was not Hattwick's concern. He was a technician's technician—knowledge for its own sake—and his success, in his eyes, was independent of the program's. Quoting our interview again: "What mattered to us was knowing exactly what was going on. That's how *we* measured success."

Third, state plans were solicited and reviewed in quick time. CDC wanted above all to get the states started on recruiting staff, procuring guns for fast injection, and ironing out details rapidly enough so that the immunization could at least begin during July. In CDC itself much work was done on educational materials for local use, a form of technical assistance. But CDC could not lay down the infrastructure for immunization. Local conditions had to be allowed to govern how the vaccinations would actually be conducted. CDC could only defray extra costs and offer free advice; it did not try to impose tight standards on state plans.

While this was happening in CDC, Cavanaugh, from the White House, reflecting Ford's commitment and his own involvement, watched the evolution of the whole program. His recollection, as he told us, is that:

Mathews felt responsible for the program, Cooper wanted to run it, and Sencer was determined to do so out of CDC. Their jockeying delayed getting the thing off the ground and especially delayed coming to grips with liability.

. . . The basic elements of the program that were operating out of CDC got off to a swift start, notably state plans and other aspects of Millar's operation. Up above, where CDC met the Assistant Secretary and the Assistant Secretary met the Secretary, it looked more confused than perhaps it really was. . . .

The Domestic Council sought and got first weekly, then bi-weekly, status reports from Meriwether. These were supplemented by occasional calls to Cavanaugh or Johnson, as matters arose requiring their intervention with other departments. As the spring wore on, the biggest of these became liability.

With the Secretary on the sidelines, Cooper at the top, White House liaison arranged, and CDC or BoB doing the work, internal organization from mid-April on was relatively clear, even coherent, as perceived inside the program, and apparently as seen from the state capitols. It was less so as seen from Capitol Hill; indeed Chairman Rogers, aware of early jockeying and soon to be beset by liability, recalls "disorganization" as the most disturbing feature of the whole affair. "There were too many cooks, no clear line of command, no single 'head' to hold responsible or ask for information." In this he sees *the* lesson for next time.

Rogers almost certainly reads summer troubles back into the spring. He said to us:

Ted Cooper is a very able person. It struck me that he knew what he was doing and trying hard. But every so often Mathews got into the situation. Sometimes I couldn't tell who was in charge—Cooper, Mathews or Taft [William Howard Taft IV, the new HEW General Counsel, who became involved during the summer]. Cooper often didn't have as much authority as he should have.

On the Senate side, Chairman Kennedy has comparable recollections. These strike us as a tribute to Cooper's congressional relations: Inside he appeared a strong man, "Big Doctor," "Substitute Secretary," in the words of two associates, while on the Hill he seemed a good man beset by Mathews.

Actually, whatever else he may have been, Cooper was a man

dependent upon three subordinates whose long service had adjusted their relations with one another, Sencer, Meyer and Seal. Adjustments had been careful: accommodations among equals, gentlemen's agreements. Cooper might be the boss, but they ran their own agencies and their agreements more than his intentions set the swine flu program's course.

6

FIELD TRIALS

On March 25, the day after the President's announcement, a meeting chaired by Meyer at the BoB—with CDC and NIAID and the producing laboratories represented—drew several key conclusions. These had been in the air March 10 or even earlier; this meeting tacked them down.

First, manufacturers should produce enough swine vaccine for everyone—roughly 200 million doses—and start deliveries in June for use from July on. Neither now nor later were dates for the mass immunization made precise. The aim was to start before August—as early in July as deliveries allowed—and to finish before winter. (In their April testimony, Sencer and Cooper said November; whereas Meyer, closer to production, said late December.)

Second, since this would fully occupy available facilities of active manufacturers, no more Victoria vaccine should be produced. What was at hand would be made bivalent by adding swine vaccine in bulk. This would produce some 30 million bivalent doses, to be used for high-risk groups, mainly the elderly.

Third, the rest of the swine flu vaccine would be turned into monovalent doses and used on a one-person, one-dose basis, thus insuring wide availability. This assumed that one dose would give adequate protection without bothersome effects on adults and children alike. The assumption was colored by recent improvements in vaccine purification. But it rested fundamentally on logistical concerns: how could one hope to get vaccine and kids together twice?

Fourth, the needs of the armed forces, also those of the VA, although separately determined and contracted for (as usual), had to fit inside these targets, with deliveries coordinated in a fashion to which military doctors were distinctly unaccustomed. Production orders from still other sources, including other countries if they came, had to wait upon American deliveries. Diversions of American supplies would be a matter for the White House (so indeed was the compliance of DoD: Cavanaugh later got stuck with both).

Another assumption was hidden, or more precisely muffled, in these calculations, namely that the manufacturers would grow the monovalent vaccine fast enough to guard against an early fall pandemic. In 1918, the virulent phase had begun in August. The manufacturers now argued, in Hilleman's words at the meeting:

> . . . you couldn't possibly have 200 million doses by fall. . . . If you are talking about one dose per egg, which is more what it looks like [instead of the hoped-for two doses] you are talking about a different situation.[6]

The day before, the President had pledged vaccine to everyone. A week later, Cooper, on the Hill, would state his goal as "95 percent of all Americans." Hilleman's discrepancy seems to have left Meyer untroubled.

On April 2, Sencer in Atlanta hosted a monster meeting to acquaint state health officials and representatives of private medicine with these targets (Congress willing) and with CDC's conception of administrative follow-through based on state immunization plans. Prompt filing of these plans was sought by CDC. Funding and technical assistance were to follow. Vaccine distribution would begin as soon as field trials, tests and bottling allowed, and states should start at once to put it into people.

Taking maximum advantage of the time at hand, the states now had a chance to immunize the country, or most of it, before the next flu season.

Here was a challenge for the Public Health officialdom from coast to coast, an opportunity to do in 1976 precisely what had not been done in 1968 or 1957—and at Federal expense with the President responsible. Energy and time and personnel might have to be withdrawn from other uses, to be sure, but not much money begged from any legislature except Congress; his trouble, not theirs. Besides, there was the vision of the Kilbournes and the Coopers: preventive medicine raised high in public consciousness. Who could be against that?

Actually, there seem to have been many persons present who, in some degree or other, feared the swine flu program either as a dubious diversion from less speculative ventures—measles, polio—or as a likely failure in the public mind, the opposite of Kilbourne's view, or worse, as a presumptive danger *to* the public health because of unknown side effects, the Alexander worry. Jonathan Fielding, Massachusetts Commissioner of Public Health, told us that he remembers disagreeing:

I didn't favor a mass vaccination program because I thought the risk of an epidemic small and I didn't want to divert resources from other programs.

But Massachusetts had a long-standing feud with CDC and everybody knew it.

One Regional Director of the HEW who had come to the meeting with officials from "his" states wrote afterwards:

How certain are we that an epidemic or pandemic will occur? There is a recognition that this decision [to proceed] is based on probability. Yet the recommendation to go forward was not wholly persuasive.

How certain are we that this virus will be a "killer," or possibly a "normal" virus resulting in relatively mild illness? The answer seems to be the latter. . . . This answer also relates to the relative lack of certainty that the epidemic-pandemic will occur, thus combining to weaken the threshold assertion to go forward with the program.

This might have been interesting before decision; coming after, it was taken as spectator sportsmanship.

Alexander, hearing of the meeting, wrote Sencer a tactful note:

I received the minutes of the ACIP meeting of March 10th and found them accurate and a good summary. . . . I have also seen newspaper reports of jousting with the state health officials. . . . I do not understand how practical political animals (which they should be) can be so short-sighted as not to appreciate the far bigger potential gain for the field of preventive medicine. . . .

However, my reason for writing is to say once more that I strongly recommend some hesitation before beginning vaccine administration programs. . . . I realize that there is some risk to be taken in delaying in that, like A/Victoria, we may be one of the first countries to be hit—but we may not. And most of our recent experiences with new variants—and the experience in 1918—was with a longer period of warning before the first severe wave (called the second wave in December 1918). Furthermore, although there might be some morbidity and mortality in an initial wave, there would still be some opportunity to have a major effect in dampening or preventing the second, third and other waves. And in so doing, we would have experience to guide us concerning the age distribution of severe and fatal disease.

As stated in the . . . minutes, "it was agreed that the production of vaccine must proceed and that a plan for vaccine administration must be developed." I, for one, do not agree that it need necessarily be carried out, unless there was another swine outbreak.

It is prudent and necessary to protect the population against a potential threat. . . . We spend large sums of money . . . stockpiling for military defense of the continental United States . . . with well worked-out contingency plans for use. . . .

I urge you to consider this. There still seems to be time to be cautious if there is no further evidence of significant swine outbreaks by September. Of course, if they do occur, here or in the Southern hemisphere—the subject is dead.

With personal regards from your "half-a-hog" colleague. . . .

The tone tells volumes about the relations of advisers to directors in Sencer's world.

And Goldfield blew his top. Ignoring those relations, heedless of hierarchy, he expressed his opposition in the meeting, repeated it to the inquiring press and possibly to his surprise was featured on all network TV news shows. The CBS transcript quotes him on the April 2 Evening News:

There are as many dangers to going ahead with immunizing the population as there are withholding. We can soberly estimate that approximately fifteen percent of the entire population will suffer disability reaction.[7]

Goldfield shared Alexander's view that mass immunization should not follow planning unless swine flu actually appeared again and showed itself to be more than a fluke. Unlike Alexander, Goldfield had a particular worry, the potential side effects in pregnant mothers. Sharing this with his college-aged daughter, he had been sternly urged to go public. But this specific risk, unfortunately for him, was discounted by specialists, and he with it, obscuring Alexander's general point.

Goldfield thereupon became a source of professional controversy. He was admired in some quarters for his candor and lambasted in others for disloyalty. One of the country's senior epidemiologists told us he had admonished him: "Marty, you have some good points. I agree with much of what you say. But the decision's made. Now is the time to close ranks. You are wrong to go public." That was deemed unforgivable. By all accounts, including his own, Goldfield has *not* been forgiven.

Neither have the networks. At CDC, officials still shake their heads sadly as they think of it. One commented to us:

There was 98 percent agreement with us in that audience. . . . Only a handful of people spoke on the other side. But they got more time on the screen. . . . The critics first. . . . Goldfield, of all people, had the most attention.

He also had the most impassioned manner and the special claim of coming from New Jersey. Each network balanced him with a supportive public health official from somewhere else. To us, the coverage seems both predictable and professional—professional, that is to say, in terms of news, not medicine.

CDC officials got a further jolt from the editorial page of the

New York Times. The paper's reportage was comprehensive, factual, and careful, regarded as a model in Atlanta. This made all the more painful a succession of editorials, which began by questioning and ended by denouncing the swine flu program. The first of these had come February 23, after the initial CDC press conference. The second, in a stiffer tone, came April 6, four days after CDC's meeting with the states. At CDC, there was great puzzlement about one newspaper's ability to be so courtly on the news page and so nasty on the editorial. In fact, the editorials were written by one member of the Editorial Board, Harry Schwartz, entirely on his initiative, out of his own skepticism about public medicine. As he read the news reports, the scientific case had not been made and Ford had probably been panicked.

Five days after the meeting in Atlanta, the World Health Organization held a meeting in Geneva, and CDC attendees gave a briefing on American opinions and intentions. With no recorded outbreaks anywhere else, and still only one here, their auditors kept cool (which was convenient, since they mostly lacked funds or facilities to readily follow our lead). The relative calm was reflected in a CBS Evening News story from Geneva, April 8:

> . . . preparation for a possible swine flu epidemic next winter. The Geneva experts said inoculation supplies may run short in some countries and they urged other emergency measures, including the stockpiling of vaccine.

The British set up a program for high-risk groups, along with a small stockpile, and some researchers undertook experiments with living subjects, testing the severity of the new virus. The Canadians took steps to interest their provincial health authorities in mass immunization. Unlike us, they dealt with the issue through usual channels where the provinces decide priorities in allocating limited funds. The national Health Ministry's equivalent of ACIP urged flu shots for half the population in a set of high-risk groups *excluding* healthy children and most adults between 40 and 65. The provinces acceded, scraping funds out of their regular health budgets.[8]

Meanwhile, American field trials were being planned. As

usual, NIAID, BoB, and CDC had comfortably divided up responsibility. The trials were to start as soon as funds and vaccine were available. It would be necessary to include vaccine from every manufacturer and to test the uses of both "whole" and "split" (two different methods of preparing the killed-virus vaccine). Since immunization would be on a bigger scale than ever before, there was concern to make the field trials match. The sample was to be the biggest yet, with thousands of volunteers divided into different age groups receiving different doses of vaccine from different manufacturers.

Unfortunately, the trials made no provision for checking the responses of young volunteers as between one dose or two. The program had been predicated on one dose apiece for all. It was well understood that children, lacking long exposure to related viruses, were likelier than adults to need stronger doses but to take a single dose with more discomfort. Yet one-person-one-dose was so well in mind, so much part of the program, that no one insisted on simultaneous trials of two.

Retrospectively, officials are regretful. Seal, for instance, said when interviewed:

> It would have been no trouble to bring back the volunteers in the right age groups for a second shot of split vaccine. The same subjects . . . no new selection process . . . the one consent form. . . . We just didn't think of it. . . .
> There's another lesson. . . .

Actually, it was thought of, but promptly discarded. The lesson lies in that. At the BoB meeting March 25, several outside scientists had urged inclusion of a two-dose test. The point was made, but the NIAID planners did not pick it up.

The field trials were launched April 21, with experimental lots of vaccine from the manufacturers; they for their part did what their own scientists, their laboratory specialists, said should be done. Mindful of the President's announcement, knowing that the funds had been appropriated, spurred by fellow professionals in PHS and sharing most of their concerns, the laboratories went full-tilt to meet governmental targets, rounding off Victoria while building up swine vaccine. They gambled on the field trials and counted on BoB licensing thereafter. One of them, Parke-Davis, mistakenly made several million doses of vaccine against a swine flu virus of a slightly different sort than CDC's Fort Dix strain. This was not discovered until June (and the source of the mistake, whether private lab or public, is now being judged in the courts).

Generally, production picked up smoothly though less rapidly than had been hoped in March. Low yield-per-egg was one problem. Other manufacturing impediments slowed some production labs; how much is hard to tell. Each company's vaccine is somewhat different from the others. Their products must meet the same FDA standards, but their processes are private. Taken as a whole, we know that their production rates fell below Sencer's (hence Cooper's) early expectations. Just how much and why is obscured by the privacy. The GAO Report has some suggestive data on how much. The answer to the why may be as simple as lack of realism in those expectations.

While NIAID prepared for field trials, Millar and his associates at CDC were seeking and then processing state plans. The states, along with cities which had separate health departments, offered a variety of plans. Some, like Delaware and New Jersey, were statewide; some, like California and Pennsylvania, were county-by-county (depending on state size and on the relative authority of local and state health agencies). Some sought guns for only a few roving teams; others sought to mount supplies for many. Pennsylvania and New Jersey are again in contrast. Some assumed use of the public schools (available in summer), others featured hospitals or other health facilities. Some stressed vaccination at the work place, planning a big role for corporations; others counted mainly on their public health facilities. And in a few jurisdictions, including New York City, where public health officials were most skeptical of flu, they produced plans, took the money, and postponed aggressive action until signs of a pandemic (which they doubted) should appear. One state commissioner who held back on implementation claimed to us:

We could have mass-vaccinated this state in six weeks, and would have, if the situation with swine flu had become critical. No problem. Well, sure, there are problems, but in a real emergency, volunteer help shows up. We could have gotten to everybody you could ever get to in six weeks.

We draw these characteristics from among four states and one city sampled by the GAO—Florida, Georgia, Missouri, Pennsylvania, and Philadelphia—together with some superficial sampling of our own in California, Delaware, Massachusetts, Minnesota, New Jersey, New York and Wisconsin.

While state plans were coming in, the field trials ended and evaluation began. That process took two weeks. By the time it was over some of the assumptions which the states had used (on CDC's say so) were in collapse. The evaluation implied that immunization should begin by leaving out all persons under 18, perhaps all those under 24; whether they were ever to be covered was now said to be dependent on another set of field trials. This news was particularly irritating to the many states, Pennsylvania for one, which had intended schools as immunization centers. They had to replan. The rest had to revise their estimates of need and of peak loads.

On June 21 and 22, NIAID played host in Bethesda to a joint meeting of the BoB Review Panel on Viral and Rickettsial Vaccine and the ACIP. CDC and BoB were amply represented. So were state health departments. Sabin was there; he had asked to be invited. Salk was there as well. So were doubters and detractors in observer status, Wolfe included. And the press was there in force. About 200 people came together for those days, another monster meeting—monstrous as some saw it (Sabin among them).

The purposes announced were first to brief advisers on the field trial findings, then to hear and discuss their views (with the consensus cranked up by two *ad hoc* subcommittees over lunch). Sabin had let it be known that he sought discussion also of an active form of stockpiling in lieu of the prospective immunization. In an informal way, this became the agenda item for the second day.

The story on the field trials was both simple and depressing: single doses worked poorly on children. For persons under 18, especially young children, "whole" vaccine was immunizing but caused many reactions ranging from sore arms to high fever.

For the same group "split" vaccine did nothing of the sort, but also did not immunize. The obvious answer was half-strength doses of whole vaccine, given twice, some weeks apart. Quite possibly, a second dose of "split" vaccine would do as well, but this was not established. Yet how, if a pandemic came, get children back a second time? Besides, how get enough vaccine? All production schedules had assumed one child, one dose.

Discussions of the reactivity of whole vaccine and the potency of split led to an inevitable proposal. There should be another set of field trials to establish the results of second doses. The production question could be faced, and distribution also, after that was done. Sencer soon would say to an inquiring reporter for TV:

What we're telling mothers for the next two months is that as scientists we don't know what to tell them, that we're doing the work that is going to be necessary to be able to give them good advice. And that's all we can say for the next two months because we just don't know the answers.[9]

But there also was, implicitly, a further answer. This, although not publicly acknowledged, seems to have been understood by all advisers and officials on the scene. As one of them told us:

What Sencer meant but could not say is that if a pandemic came we'd use single shots of whole vaccine on children; no matter how uncomfortable it made them, mothers wouldn't mind. But in the absence of another outbreak, and a big one, no, we couldn't use it, mothers would mind too damn much. As for the split vaccine, it was all over for 1976. We had to go through field trials first; then how could we get twice as much vaccine as we originally ordered? In time, that is, for the flu season? Maybe 1978? So we knew in June that children were out unless the flu exploded, which by then was seeming more and more remote. But we had to order up new field trials . . . and we couldn't simply say "no kids."

They couldn't because they thought most Americans, recalling polio, expected kids and shots to go together like ham and eggs. Immunization without children would sound crazy. What sort of preventive medicine was that? What sort of parental consciousness raising?

Both in what he said and in what he evidently thought, Sencer reflected the views of his colleagues.

On stockpiling, by contrast, Sencer squared off against Sabin, who if not a colleague was at least a member of the club. Sabin had come to make two points quite separate from, although enlivened by, the children's problem. He argued, first, in terms like Alexander's, the case for watchful waiting now that no swine flu had shown up anywhere, not even in the Southern Hemisphere, where flu season would shortly reach its peak. The case was only strengthened by the likelihood that we would not now immunize the children. In previous pandemics, children had been the chief spreaders of disease. And second, Sabin argued that with proper preparation we could keep ahead of spread, inoculating quickly if the virus reappeared. The form of stockpiling was to be active, not passive, not mere warehousing. Proper measures in his view included both planning and training. He called for brigades of volunteers—high school age and up—recruited and trained locally, ready to immunize their neighborhoods the moment CDC should pass the word. In the minutes:

> We must be able to do [immunize] everybody in an area in 1 to 2 days. We need a total voluntary effort, training . . . students and others in an assembly-line technique. We cannot rely on health professionals and existing doctors' offices.[10]

Sencer, armed with a brief staff study, spoke out against this course on grounds of feasibility. His assistant director for operations, Dr. William Foege, strongly seconded him. The flu could move too fast, "jet-spread" again. That CDC staff study is the only written piece of staff work we can find on stockpiling; as such we include it in Appendix D. The study's objections to stockpiling centered on timing. Among its assumptions, three were questionable. The first was that many workers would have to be newly recruited and trained in an emergency; treating the whole of emergency staff like Army reservists was not explored. The second was that emergency clinics would work on a six-day week; working on Sundays was not discussed. The third was that "commitment" to a standby program would decline over time necessarily; the adrenal charge of a perceived emergency was nowhere recognized, nor was the draining effect of doubts about the program as it stood. Even so, Sencer argued hard (and probably still would).

The ACIP minutes for June 22 reflect his and Foege's views:

> . . . the infeasibility of achieving any measure of adequate immunization of the country once cases or clusters of cases were occurring . . . once operational, most immunization programs would take two to three months to complete even if all elements functioned smoothly and personnel, vaccine supplies and other program ingredients were ample . . . once identified as causing cases, pandemic strains can be expected to become widespread in less than two months, . . . no rational basis for a general 'stockpiling concept' . . . more risk in this concept when one adds a two-week period of antibody development onto the vaccination timetable.

Sencer also stressed that high school volunteers were bait for litigation. This last was a note to which all ears were just becoming sensitive. Besides, as several state officials said, plans now had gone too far to be revised wholesale in Sabin's fashion. Projects had momentum; break it and it would not soon revive.

In the minds of some committee members this turned the argument. Stallones, for one, recalled to us:

> I had talked to Alexander, and I was impressed by his point of view, although in March I had been an enthusiast for going all the way. But what Foege said was impressive too, and to have it reinforced by the state people themselves struck me personally as compelling.

At all events, a clear majority of the combined committees went along with CDC and state desires as expressed. Along with dosage recommendations, mass immunization was reaffirmed. Storing doses in people, not warehouses, as Salk said, won the day among those voting at Bethesda. Thereafter Cooper turned to Salk as once to Sabin.

The press found much of interest in these meetings, and the television news found interesting faces to present, both old and new. Postponement of the children caused wry comment on two networks, and the stockpiling debate was featured on all three. Sabin was the Goldfield of this coverage, but he was joined by others, notably Alexander, moved by three more months without a trace of swine flu. Uncharacteristically, Alexander went public:

> I think the issue is, as time goes on, there—it's becoming more evident that up till now there's no sign of swine influenza outbreaks like the one that occurred in Fort Dix, New Jersey occurring in the United States. Most people think that the probability is there will not be an epidemic in the 1976–77 season due to swine influenza.[11]

Other opponents cited in the newspapers, or shown on the TV, included those who had appeared when the program was first announced. But this was no mere replay of initial skepticism; Sabin and Alexander demonstrated that. The point was not lost in such places as the Editorial Board of the *New York Times*, or the Washington Bureau of CBS News. Nor was it lost in Congress. Congressman Henry A. Waxman of the Rogers subcommittee, an habitual watcher of CBS News, seems to have been much struck by the whole proceeding; Senator Kennedy has told us he recalls stockpiling as an opportunity lost.

At CDC and Cooper's office, and indeed in Cavanaugh's, reactions against Sabin (who had been so eloquently their man on TV three months ago) remind us of White House reactions against favored columnists who come up with what staffers take as slurs upon their President. But White House aides, more royalist than the king, grow angry in defending *him*. The health officials here, excepting Cavanaugh, were not concerned with Ford. Their anger was indeed aroused but they defended something else: as best we can discern, it was the sanctity of hierarchical decisions in their profession. They are scornful of Sabin yet. Alexander they merely cold-shouldered.

And the media in their view had distorted once again, with emphasis on controversy rather than agreement.

However, these officials did not have much time, just then, to dwell upon past grievances. For they were being threatened from another quarter. The Bethesda meetings were scarcely adjourned when word came that the casualty insurance industry could find no members willing to insure the manufacturers of swine vaccine. The manufacturers refused to bottle it until somebody did.

7

LIABILITY

On June 25, Leslie Cheek, chief of the Washington branch office of the American Insurance Association, made a courtesy call to Meriwether, Meyer and Sencer, among others, on a conference hook-up. He told them what he'd spent a week determining in calls around the casualty industry, which AIA represented. The manufacturers of swine vaccine would not get liability insurance. Liability potential was enormous and, worse, uncertain. The necessary underwriting could not be arranged. Existing coverage would terminate June 30, for all manufacturers. Meyer was incredulous. Sencer laughed wryly. Meriwether's reaction is not recorded.

For at least a month, they and their HEW colleagues had known they were in trouble. On May 24, counsel for Merrell, one of the manufacturers, had broken off six weeks of contract negotiations, insisting on indemnification by the government for most prospective legal costs associated with the swine flu program. Reluctantly HEW counsel had drafted and the OMB, still more reluctantly, had approved an indemnification bill. On June 15 the Chairman of Parke-Davis, another manufacturer, had wired all and sundry that it stood to lose insurance coverage

June 30. This at once became public, which did nothing to enhance the reputation of swine flu vaccine.

The bill had gone to Congress June 16. Its reception had been cool. Neither on the Hill nor in the Public Health Service had threatened loss of coverage been taken literally. Nothing like that had ever occurred with immunization programs.

So June 25 was a shock. Suddenly, the immunization program—just reaffirmed at Bethesda—seemed wholly dependent on congressional action in a complicated field, not previously explored, six weeks before the scheduled recess for Ford's still uncertain nomination. Following Merrell's lead, all manufacturers made plain that they would not insure themselves, not even temporarily. Instead they put off plans to bottle their vaccine; pending legislation they would keep the stuff in bulk. Each week's delay in moving from bulk to bottles assured at least as much delay in starting inoculations. Thus ended hopes of immunizing *any*body in July or even August.

The question becomes, why did the Government proceed into June without facing this eventuality? The question is important. The answer takes us back to liability as seen in PHS before Fort Dix. And then we must retrace some steps from January to June.

Liability for vaccine-related injury had been a tender topic with the drug manufacturers since the early 1960's, when the courts had first begun to hand down adverse judgments. The cases were still rare then, most stemming from polio immunization, but the awards were large and the trend unsettling. In 1974 the problem ballooned in the case of *Reyes* v. *Wyeth* (498 F2nd 1264). Wyeth was another vaccine manufacturer. The circuit court upheld a jury award of $200,000 to an eight-month-old infant who had contracted polio after receiving Sabin live-virus vaccine. The Supreme Court refused to hear the case; the award held. Wyeth had failed to extend an adequate warning of the risk of harm to the unlucky vaccinee. Never mind that the company had included in cartons for shipment a printed form which *did* contain adequate warning. Never mind that experts had testified at trial that this particular case was not vaccine-related. Wyeth would pay (and did). The suffering was real and Wyeth had the only deep pocket available.

To BoB and CDC, concerned for an assured vaccine supply, the inference drawn from *Reyes* had been that if the government proposed to sponsor mass immunizations, but not to make vaccine itself, it must take over the duty to warn, opening *its* pocket, or indemnify the private firms, or compensate victims directly. The manufacturers were eager to unload the *Reyes* duty. In their eyes it was a quite unreasonable cost of doing business. In the eyes of Sencer's staffers, also many of Meyer's and Seal's, it was a cost of doing business that the manufacturers could all too easily avoid by dropping vaccines from their product lines. So at these staff levels there was a coincidence of interest with the private firms, premised on need for relief from the duty to warn.

At various times staff papers on the subject went to Cooper with no result. In January 1976, just before Fort Dix, the most elaborate of these was sent forward by Sencer as a draft proposal from Cooper to Mathews. Prepared by Sencer's Assistant Director for Programs, Bruce Dull, it urged Federal indemnification wherever there was Federal sponsorship for immunization. The cover memo argued:

> Manufacturer liability for vaccine-associated disability . . . threatens a predictable vaccine supply. . . .
>
> A decision on the Secretary's part to pursue legislation for public management of vaccine-associated disability would relieve the apprehension and anxiety of public health and medical professionals and of biologics producers.

This memorandum may not have reached Cooper, much less Mathews, for it ran afoul of adverse views in Cooper's staff. The issue had been up before, positions had hardened. As an opponent recalled for our benefit:

> Behind these arguments for indemnification there were a number of assumptions which were untested and unsupported by facts. For one, it was contended that if the manufacturers were not indemnified, they would all stop making vaccine. But the number of companies in this business had been diminishing for a long time, for reasons totally unrelated to liability.
>
> We just couldn't buy this—that continued liability would drive them out.

And there were other unsupported assumptions, just sort of out there, loping across the plains.

But more than a distaste for coddling manufacturers was working at the top of PHS. There also was concern about ramifications far beyond the immunization field. Indemnification for companies (or even compensation to victims) here could be a precedent almost across the board of public health programs. These were the cautious views of Donald Carmody, an office director on Cooper's staff, professionally a lawyer, who played in-house skeptic about liability proposals. A year before Dull's memorandum, BoB had sent up somewhat comparable proposals. One of Meyer's aides had noted then:

Any provision for a Federal fund to provide such compensation will meet with objections from H, whether it be through amendment of the Federal Tort Claims Act, or, as CDC is attempting, through amendment of the PHS Act.

Carmody himself told us he thought the "H" meant him.

Beyond issues of substance and precedent were strong instincts on Cooper's part for steering clear of questions where doctors were at the mercy of lawyers. One of his close associates remarked to us:

As for lawyers, doctors think lawyers are a pain in the ass. Cooper's mind set was to keep lawyers out if you don't want it screwed up.

All this was before the swine flu program. When the manufacturers were asked to make 200 million doses by the Federal government, for Federal purchase, distributed with Federal help, for use at Federal urging in a national campaign, then Federal assumption of the duty to warn became a price one had to be prepared to pay, even in Cooper's view. Assumption of the duty did not seem to him synonymous with reimbursement for all legal costs, to say nothing of compensation for all victims. Rather, it seemed a separable and more modest concession.

Neither Cooper nor Sencer made much of this with Mathews or with Ford, nor did they try to calculate the program's added cost if *Reyes* awards resulted. They seemed to have expected that the duty to warn, once they assumed it, would be discharged too well for penalties. CDC could draw a good consent form and the vaccine, after all, was safe. As for defending against baseless suits, attorneys would be charged to other budgets than their own, in other fiscal years, no problem for the swine flu supplemental.

Preparing to brief Ford, March 22, Dickson, on Cooper's behalf, had talked at Mathews' staff meeting with St. John Barrett, HEW's Deputy General Counsel. Barrett was acting for Taft, the new General Counsel not yet confirmed. Barrett had a word with Bernard Feiner, the career head of his Business and Administrative Law Division. Meanwhile Cavanaugh, on his own motion, called Attorney General Levi, who referred him to Neil Peterson, head of Tort Claims at Justice. Peterson, Feiner and Barrett all reacted alike; the duty to warn could be carried in the government's procurement contract. This was what Cooper and Cavanaugh wanted to hear. It spared them going, hat in hand, to the Rogers and Kennedy subcommittees for substantive legislation, which might slow appropriations and delay the program's start. Comparatively speaking, it was better to go to the lawyers: Cooper did so. Mathews approved. Cavanaugh did not demur. The problem did not figure in the issues put to Ford, and landed in the lap of OGC.

No part of HEW was less prepared to cope with liability than was the General Counsel's Office. In form it has a vast array of lawyers, in fact a handful who are not absorbed by endless streams of regulation-writing, bill-drafting, contracting or litigating. The number of able attorneys free to tackle tedious and complicated issues without deadlines, lacking pressure from the Secretary, or equivalent, was virtually nil in Barrett's time—and is so still. Nobody had fastened on a problem which a Dull could not get past a Carmody.

Now, however, with a novel form of contract to contrive, Barrett had to improvise. He turned to Feiner because contracts were familiar in the Business Division's work. And Feiner took the task upon himself because, as one of his superiors told us: "He was a good lawyer, meticulous . . . and the only one in the division competent to do it."

Thus Dull's interest in duty to warn survived his paper and

was carried by swine flu momentum to the HEW lawyers. But it was stripped of Dull's original concern about production. After all, the manufacturers could scarcely stop producing in the middle of a national program. Swine flu momentum would carry them, too, along with the issue and even despite it.

That is how Cavanaugh, Cooper and Mathews seem to have reasoned and how Barrett and Feiner proceeded, from March through May.

Unfortunately, assuming the duty to warn through contract provisions failed to satisfy the manufacturers. The government could undertake to warn. But suppose the manufacturers should be sued anyway. Suppose the courts should sympathize, enlarging *Reyes*. Awards aside, what of the legal costs to cope with baseless suits? While legal overhead would pass to casualty insurers above a self-insurance limit, might there not be more than enough suits to crowd that limit? Manufacturers accepted their responsibility for simple negligence, but these questions ranged far beyond negligence to an uncharted realm suggested by absolute liability, 200 million doses, friendly juries, and the itch to sue. Yet contract language could not assure indemnity for anything. The Anti-Deficiency Act stood in the way. It barred agency spending without statutory sanction. The courts long since had said this meant no open-ended promises by such as HEW.

Barrett and Feiner, with help from Justice, sought contract language that would stretch the limits of that Act. Washington counsel for three of the four manufacturers joined in with dubiety. As one of them put it to us:

We would open every meeting with a heartfelt refrain for the HEW lawyers: "We need legislative relief. Nothing short of that is going to do it. [Chairman] Rogers would be willing to put in a bill. We need legislative relief." That was our first paragraph at every session. It fell on absolutely deaf ears. We would watch it fall, and then we would proceed to talk about what they wanted to talk about.

What counsel stressed in their opening comments did not seem to be what their clients were stressing in public statements to others. The clients spoke mainly of duty to warn. Joseph

Stetler, President of the Pharmaceutical Manufacturers Association in Washington, had twice testified on the Hill; when it came to liability, he asked for indemnification, but he emphasized shifting the duty imposed by *Reyes*:

. . . Wyeth was sued, held responsible, and told they had the responsibility to advise every person being immunized of potential harm and danger from the vaccine. This is an absolutely impossible requirement, particularly if you are talking about a nationwide immunization program. It is that kind of precedent that makes us very properly concerned about our potential liability under this program. It is a responsibility that is going to have to be shared by the Government in this unusual partnership arrangement we find ourselves in.

By mid-May, Feiner's work on contract language had brought all concerned as far as there seemed any point in going. It may be that the counsel for the three firms would have urged agreement on their clients, trusting to the good will of the government if catastrophic costs were actually incurred. Barrett and Feiner were hopeful then; our interviews suggest they had some reason.

But on May 24, counsel for the fourth firm, Merrell, called a halt. William Rogers, the former Secretary of State, came in as senior counsel to pronounce the word. Merrell would not proceed without assurance of indemnification, except for negligence.

Barrett went to Cooper with a question: Did the program really need Merrell's production? Cooper consulted Sencer and then took the answer to Mathews. On their March assumptions it had to be yes. Nothing had changed those assumptions. Merrell was the smallest of the firms but had been scheduled for a quarter of the swine flu production. Reluctantly they acquiesced, as Cavanaugh and O'Neill did in turn, to what the firms and CDC had wanted from the start, an indemnification bill.

Behind Merrell's firmness, there almost certainly was fear of the intentions of the casualty insurers. In May it was no secret that at least some major firms wanted to steer clear of swine vaccine. As early as April 8, Merck had been warned by its primary insurer that coverage for swine vaccine was "considered" not "feasible . . . at virtually any price." So Merck's President had written Mathews and everyone else in sight.[12] Merrell, then about to switch insurers (for unrelated reasons), is reported to have been told by its new one something of the same sort at about the same time. We do not know precisely what was made of this, where, in Merrell's management. We do know that the issue was reviewed again, in June, by the insurer with the same result, a "no." But we assume that Merrell's counsel knew in May what the insurer had already warned in April. However that may be, it shortly would turn out that all insurers saw the swine flu program much alike: *not* for them.

Insurance managements apparently were concerned less with duty to warn and court awards than with that other spectre, overhead costs. Their eyes were fixed on claims and beyond these on law suits. Under prevailing contracts with drug companies, the primary insurers were obliged to defend them in court. Granting the potential for some catastrophic losses, in between awards were all the suits to be dismissed. How many cases, how many lawyers, how much time, what cost? 200 million doses meant how many million claims to overstrain adjusters? Poorly adjusted claims would turn into how many million lawsuits? Suits are fueled by anger. Governmental urging meant how many angry citizens? Would Presidential sponsorship, hence "politics" in an election year, anger them still more? This we are told weighed heavily. And back of anger, what might be the side effects to give it verisimilitude and lengthen legal process?

These questions defied actuaries. There was no experience. Polio immunization had entailed far fewer numbers with sponsorship free from political taint, in a relatively unlitigious era. The upshot was too much uncertainty for managements like these to bear. They were just coming out of a two-year financial squeeze. They were in business to spread risk, not take it. What they couldn't calculate could not be spread on any terms they cared for. Nor could the primary insurers unload costs of their adjusters and house counsel.

For the insurers, Ford's announcement raised a red flag. Cheek, a Washington lawyer, not previously much exposed to the internal management concerns of those he represented there, has speculated to us:

I wouldn't be surprised if some president or senior vice-president in each company hadn't happened to catch Ford on the evening news and said to himself: "Every man, woman, and child! I wonder if we cover any of the vaccine manufacturers—if we do, we certainly ought to cancel."

The President of one of the companies smiles at this. He told us:

It may be so for the others, but in our case it was some junior underwriters who noticed first. Their worry was "how would a catastrophic award look on my record?" The thing worked its way up. . . . The higher it got, the more it was seen in the broader management context, claims and suits: incalculable amounts of overhead cost for which we had unlimited liability. Our Vice President . . . decided not to insure. Then he put his decision to me, which he usually wouldn't do, because of the White House announcement, the public affairs aspect. I simply confirmed his decision. . . . If the public was really endangered, the government should take the risk; it certainly could, we couldn't.

Whichever way decision-making moved, top-down or bottom-up, Cheek would not have known it then. He ran but a branch office for his trade association, watching Congress and explaining why his clients couldn't cover natural disasters. The casualty insurance industry was regulated by the states. It had no Federal agency with which it dealt from day to day, least of all HEW.

Some firms that sold casualty insurance also sold health insurance, but the work was compartmentalized internally, and governmental contracts were facilitated through separate trade associations. The AIA, Cheek's outfit, had its headquarters in New York, with many branches, of which his was only one. But as he saw it from afar, to quote our interview again:

If top management asked about particular coverage, it would take about two weeks for the inquiry to get down to the underwriters concerned and come back up. There would be nothing much else for the top to do except in due course to pass the word back, "When the contracts re-open, don't renew."

If decisions flowed the other way the timing might be shorter.

On April 12, Cheek's boss T. Lawrence Jones came down from New York for a meeting with Lynn on another subject. At the end they had some words on swine flu liability. At AIA it is considered that Lynn then got a forewarning of the uninsurability of swine vaccine. If so, it did not register sufficiently to be passed on. OMB staff do not recall it. Neither does O'Neill or Cavanaugh. And nobody from AIA called Cooper or Barrett.

No aspect of the swine flu case holds more intrinsic interest than the solid wall between decision processes at HEW, on the one hand, and the insurance managements on the other. The drug company managements were somewhere in the middle. How much they knew by when about their prospects for insurance is unclear to us. The chain is long. At one end was the Washington counsel negotiating with Barrett, next were house counsel and top management of manufacturing subsidiaries, next their counterparts at corporate headquarters, then (in three cases out of four) headquarters specialists in insurance placement, then the outside brokers with whom they dealt, and finally the insurance underwriters heading up to their own managements. And it was not one chain but five, in parallel, from four drug companies to five primary insurers (one of the drug companies was shifting its insurance). Who knew what, when, along these chains, to say nothing of across them, we can only conjecture.

Two things, however, strike us now. First, nobody had incentives to assume the worst except those farthest away from HEW, the insurance managements. Everybody else had incentives to hope for the best. Second, at no time before June did HEW attempt to find or deal directly with its opposite numbers, the insurance managements. Who was to do that? Why? HEW dealt with the manufacturers. As Mathews later told the press:

The insurance companies are parties to the manufacturers, not to us. We are not in direct negotiations with them except through the manufacturers. . . .

The issue is between them and their manufacturers . . . not between them and us. . . .[13]

Cooper now considers this a lesson to be learned; he told us:

If I had it to do over again, I would have talked to the insurance industry directly and not through the drug manufacturers, and I wouldn't have waited too long to start doing it. That's an important lesson.

And Mathews has a retrospective warning for us:

Mass immunization was like sending the big trucks over an old bridge; the supporting structure was not strong enough to hold up. The liability issue, and behind that, the growing litigiousness of the times, were simply too much.

By that light Cooper's lesson should be underlined. Whenever an unprecedented venture is in prospect HEW officials ought to ask themselves, "What private decision-makers (or public, for that matter) about whom we know nothing can be critical in implementing *our* decision?"—then go learn something about them.

Failure to do that cannot quite explain why CDC's identification of the liability problem, having been held down for so long, was then embraced without a hard look at its terms. The doctors drew from *Reyes* what we now know to have been too narrow a lesson, concentrating too much on the cost of awards stemming from duty to warn. The manufacturers drew a wider lesson; what might the courts pin on them next? The insurers drew a lesson wider still: verdicts aside, count up the claims, still more the suits! In OGC the implications were resisted or ignored for three months.

8

LEGISLATION

Congress gave short shrift to HEW's indemnification bill. The House Health Subcommittee held a hearing June 28, with the drug companies and HEW, as well as Cheek. Cooper was questioned hard. The companies got little sympathy. Nobody but they liked indemnification, not even the Administration witnesses. There was a smell of rip-off in the air.

WAXMAN. Dr. Cooper, are you in effect saying that the insurance industry is using the possibility of a swine flu pandemic as an excuse to blackmail the American people into paying higher insurance rates?

COOPER. Well. . . .

WAXMAN. You suggest that you don't understand why they are charging three or four times more than is customary.

COOPER. I do not. . . .

WAXMAN. It's your view that the insurance industry is not acting responsibly when they are asking to charge three or four times the usual rate for a vaccine that does not offer significant risk, while at the same time they are insuring vaccination programs where there are more substantial risks involved.[14]

Congressman Andrew Maguire of New Jersey joined his colleague Waxman in sharp questioning. They took it that there had to be some other, better way and that it would soon show itself with more intensive bargaining and higher level pressure. This was a message for Mathews. Chairman Rogers underscored it. He told Taft, who had entered the scene in Barrett's temporary absence, to get back to the bargaining table and work the thing out by contract.

Cheek recalls, as he told us:

> The subcommittee did not understand why insurers were reluctant to insure a vaccine whose medical risks appeared minimal; they certainly did not sympathize with the industry, or with our argument that the incalculable number of spurious claims and new liability doctrines made the manufacturers uninsurable at any price. . . . They just didn't believe us.

In the first week of July, the manufacturers and OGC restaged their dialogue. The stakes were higher, the publicity greater, the players more prominent, but the game was essentially the same. Feiner stretched the proffered contract language a bit more and Taft cleared it with Justice:

> D. If any claim or action by a third party is asserted against the Contractor [manufacturer] arising in whole or in part from an alleged failure by the Government properly to discharge the responsibilities assumed by it in this Article, the Contractor shall promptly notify the contracting officer. . . . The government shall, at its option, either defend against or assist in the defense or settlement of such claim. . . .
>
> E. In the event of the Government's breach of, or failure to carry out, its responsibilities . . . any measure of resulting damages to the Contractor shall include, but need not be limited to, damages (including money judgments . . . and reasonable attorneys' fees . . .) sustained in connection with claims against the Contractor caused by the breach or failure.[15]

Counsel for the manufacturers expressed themselves as nearly satisfied and talked to the insurers on July 9. But the latter's representatives were not so sanguine. They found protection still inadequate; besides, to the extent the clause *did* satisfy, it violated the spirit if not the letter of the Anti-Deficiency Act.

Mathews thereupon insisted that executives of the insurance firms meet with the manufacturers and him. They did so July

13, in his office. The drug companies took a friendly stance which they could well afford; the insurers were firm. Some observers now believe that Mathews could have budged them had he locked the door, with cameras just outside, and kept them there until they compromised. He scoffs at this. The insurance representatives were not at the right level. Besides, by July 13 his lawyers had found merit in their argument. He soon left the meeting for Cooper to run. Nothing of substance occurred. Mathews met instead with congressional staff: legislation now was of the essence again. Afterwards he called in the press: ". . . the question which has been paramount in these discussions [is] . . . who pays for suits that prove to be baseless? That is the point of great concern in this matter. . . ."

Mathews then made a date with the President. They met July 19. In preparation for that meeting Cooper sent the Domestic Council an options paper longer, more varied, and calmer in tone than Sencer's action-memorandum of four months before. We find nothing to suggest that it had any influence on Cavanaugh, O'Neill or Ford.

What influenced Ford was a simple answer to a simple question. He met with Mathews, Cavanaugh and Cooper and asked Cooper, as they all recall, if anything had changed since March in their assumptions about the disease. Cooper told him no: a pandemic remained "possible," with probabilities "unknown." The lack of cases since changed neither term. In fact, that lack had changed the feelings of most specialists who sensed that odds were dropping week by week. But there can be no fall-off from "unknown." So Cooper was correct. For Ford this was conclusive. The program must continue; he decided that it should. Congress had to be brought back into the act and he would help with that.

After the meeting Ford talked to the press:

. . . we are going to find a way, either with or without the help of Congress, to carry out this program that is absolutely essential, a program that was recommended to me unanimously by 25 or 30 of the top medical people in this particular field.[16]

He also asked Mathews to call Congressman Rogers and to draft him a letter for Rogers, which Cavanaugh actually did. Ford sent it July 23, in time for a new set of hearings.

There is no excuse to let this program, a program that could affect the lives of many, many Americans, bog down in petty wrangling. Let's work together to get on with the job.

On July 20 and again on the 23rd Rogers held more hearings. These evidently were intended to give Mathews more clout. They were aimed at the insurers' heads. This time, at Rogers' insistence, the primary insurers were represented by their own executives. Maguire and Waxman had at them with a will, and Rogers in his nice way too, all of it televised, with snippets on the network news.

Under severe pressure, the insurers promised Rogers what they had not given Mathews, a price tag on coverage for swine flu liability. Days later they presented both to Rogers and to Mathews three separate proposals for insurance pools. Only one was a complete package, and it was wildly priced. When manufacturers expressed some interest anyway, its sponsors promptly found that they could not get enough underwriting for their own plan. They were able to get the "first" level of potential costs covered (for high fees) by domestic companies, but neither at home nor abroad did they find subscribers for the "excess" level built into their plan. That was a level of potential loss per manufacturer above $12.5 million. As one of our informants said, "The excess market abandoned us."

On July 30 the insurers reverted to their previous stance. There were *no* terms on which their industry could cover liability for manufacturers of swine vaccine.

Mathews, disgusted, told Cooper and Taft to make another try for legislation. Rogers, disheartened, joined in. His subcommittee staff director, a public health professional, Dr. Lee Hyde, took leadership in looking for a substitute to indemnification. Attention came to rest on a device which had been used at HUD, an adaptation of the Tort Claims Act. But Congress was due to recess in two weeks. Prospects for action were dim.

Prospects were not improved by a subsidiary theme of subcommittee hearings two days earlier. The vaccine manufacturers had told what they were doing in the absence of insurance. They were producing only in bulk. 100 million doses sat in vats, unpooled, unbatched, unvialed and unlabeled. To go from bulk to doses in the hands of immunizers would take weeks. If nothing moved another step without new legislation, when (if ever) would inoculations start? Cooper and Sencer had once said these should *end* in November. Moreover, all around the world there had not been a single case of swine flu for six months. What were the arguments for legislating *now* some form of special benefit for insurance and drug companies? Symbolically, only oil companies could have been worse.

The answer to that question came out of the blue. On August 1 the press began reporting a new respiratory disease in Pennsylvania. By August 2 it was named "Legionnaire's Disease"; all of its victims had been at an American Legion State Convention. The disease was severe; there were deaths. The press began a body count. The TV covered funerals. And for four days swine flu seemed a possible cause. On August 5, the CDC announced its lab reports: whatever this might be, it was not that. By then legislation was well on its way to enactment. Even if this were not swine flu, a swine outbreak might well be just as photogenic.

Sencer had once put a gun to Ford's head; now events did the same to Congress.

The immediate beneficiary was the legislative formula Taft, Hyde and their associates had chanced upon. Using the Tort Claims Act as a model, Congress could specify that any claim arising from the swine flu program should be filed against the Federal government, while preserving the government's right to sue for compensation from other participants.

There was no need to "indemnify." Manufacturers were freed from the duty to warn, at least in the first instance, while they and the insurers both were freed from overhead cost: civil servants would process the claims and defend against groundless suits. With luck the insurers might never go to court at all. With still more luck they could insure the manufacturers against sheer negligence and then have none arise, thus pocketing the premiums (which did, in the event, amount to $8.5 million).

A swine flu tort claims bill, so called, drafted in a weekend, went to the House and Senate August 1. Its subsequent progress was extraordinary, testifying partly to the news, partly to Rogers' devotion. His subcommittee held a mark-up session the next day, approved the measure, and passed it along to the full House Commerce Committee. One observer's recollection helps explain Rogers' persistence: "During the mark-up, Lee Hyde kept telling stories about 1918. He believed in it; he thought it was coming. As late as that, he was deeply concerned. . . ." On August 5, however, with swine flu no longer the culprit in Philadelphia and passage no longer a matter of grave urgency, the committee chose to sit on the bill. There weren't many Hydes around. Only one week remained before Congress would quit for the Republican Convention. Ford was concerned and said so:

> HEW Secretary Mathews and the leaders of Congress reported to me Wednesday that after long hours of hearings, discussions, negotiations, Congress finally would act yesterday to pass legislation to provide swine flu vaccine to all the American people. Needless to say, I was keenly disappointed to learn last evening that the news from the doctors in Pennsylvania had led to another slowdown in the Congress.
>
> I am frankly very dumbfounded. . . .[17]

The Senate remained. Rogers and Hyde appealed to their opposite numbers. Chairman Kennedy responded. He disliked acting on a novel measure in such haste but felt he had no choice. On August 6 his subcommittee held a short hearing and voted approval; the Senate adopted a resolution sending the bill directly to the floor. On the weekend of August 7–8, HEW aides and legislative staffers hovered over the bill, squeezing in favorite provisions catch as catch can. Meanwhile, insurers slapped together plans to correspond with the protection they could now foresee. On August 10, after Rogers had failed once again to spring his own bill, the Senate acted on its version by voice vote and sent it to the House.

The President then intervened by phone and pressed the Speaker for a no-amendment rule. The Speaker called the Chairman of the Rules Committee, who acquiesced on grounds akin to national security. "Don't tell me anything about it. I don't want to know," he reportedly responded to a skeptical colleague. That was the mood in the Hall of the House. The Senate bill was rushed there without even copies for members.

It was voted three to one. Ford signed it (PL 94-380) with alacrity on August 12.

Thus the swine flu program was saved. Ford, Rogers, Mathews, Cavanaugh and Cooper, maybe Sencer, surely Taft the late arrival, were each in his way pleased, a hard task done, a purpose carried through; at last an open door to immunization. One or two levels down in PHS and CDC, a thrill went through some of the troops. Hattwick and company raced to be ready. Epidemiologists stiffened at their posts. Some others, however, were secretly sorry. For numbers of those who now had dirty work to do, coping with disgruntled states, fending off a captious press, making a late start on a no-longer-shiny program (and discounting a pandemic, as by now many did), the prospect of congressional inaction had been soothing, the more so the closer it came. By no fault of their own, they would be prevented from doing their duty—or, put another way, from doing the overblown thing their bosses had gotten them into. In ten days' time the prospect had been snatched away. Now they had to do it. Their reaction was "Oh, shit."

9

STARTING AND

STOPPING

The terms on which the swine flu program had been rescued thereupon assured that nobody could get a shot before October 1, if then. This was not instantly apparent at the White House, or to Cooper, for that matter, but it should have been. Under congressional budget procedure, the new legislation became effective with the start of the new fiscal year. Until then, manufacturers and their insurers were determined that nobody would use swine vaccine on anybody. Production and distribution proceeded accordingly. Indeed it took a lot of pleas and promises to get enough deliveries before October 1 so immunization then could make a halting start.

Like it or not, this enforced interval afforded CDC a chance to carry through in style a number of administrative chores. Both with the manufacturers and with the states there was a lot of buttoning up to do and seven weeks to do it in. But Sencer's agency seems to have been all thumbs in this respect. Our inquiry is not definitive; what it suggests, however, is that CDC, though excellent at other things, was way over its head as an administrative center for a national program.

Three examples stake out the dimensions of the problem.

First is the matter of consent forms. As part of Millar's

planning, spurred by Dull's awareness, CDC had written, printed and sent forward to the states some 60 million forms for use when vaccine was ready. Then the August legislation came along with a proviso, authored in the Kennedy Subcommittee, that a wholly separate body, the National Commission for the Protection of Human Subjects, should review and consult on consent forms. Already aggravated by delays, Sencer was furious, displaying a self-righteousness that some of his staff emulated. He reportedly announced, "I'll consult if they tell me I have to and then I'll do just what I want." This, in effect, is what happened. The National Commission was hard to assemble in August. When it did meet it was moderately critical. In retrospect its criticisms appear reasonable. Some were ignored. Others were slapped on top of CDC's form to make a two-page stapled document, with one page different for bivalent and monovalent shots. This was a messy product, hard to follow. We include it in Appendix D. Sencer and his people felt themselves unable, and certainly were unwilling, to toss out their 60 million and start over. They pleaded lack of time.

Second is the matter of manufacturers' profits. The August legislation had barred profits on swine vaccine sold to the government (although allowing them on Victoria vaccine since that had been originally intended for the market). In a statute which had government absorbing the risks for profitable companies, this limit on their profits was of obvious importance, symbolically and otherwise, to many members of Congress. CDC was the contracting agency. $100 million worth of vaccine was by its standards a huge contract. Its contract office evidently lacked either the experience or the autonomy to frame provisions which could help police those profits (at best a problematic task). Nor were CDC-ers close enough to Congress to appreciate the symbolism. The administrative judgment—quickly made, so we are told—was that time was too short for fuss; post-audit would suffice. This left the symbols in prospective disarray, and since has drawn sharp questions from the Rogers subcommittee.[18]

Third is another contract problem, the amounts and timing of vaccine deliveries. Here the contract officers, plodding a straight and narrow path, made an egregious error in external relations. They did it the day after Ford had signed his legislation. By wire to the manufacturers, they cut in half (from 100 to 50 million) their minimum purchase guarantee on swine flu doses. And they set December 3 as the last date for deliveries. The theory, at least about the date, was defensible, given the lateness of the program's start and the imminence of flu season. The symbolism was intolerable, given Ford's and Cooper's pledges that there would be shots for everyone. Predictably the manufacturers protested, Sencer retorted, Mathews urged speed and Ford got sore: "That program damn well better run right."[19] Then Rogers held a hearing, the manufacturers made a case, Cooper overruled Sencer, and the deadline was extended to January 15. The cumulative total of swine doses would then be 146 million, enough for everyone over 18, however belated their shots.

Up the hill and down again. What was the point in all that?

Sencer, defending the performance of his people, told us that in these instances they were the prisoners of Feiner's lawyers and of local counsel who compounded indecisiveness with nitpicking. If so, two staffs in combination failed to cope with the dimensions of the work they had to do.

With each of these examples, the press could have had quite a lot of fun had not Ford's nomination and the start of the campaign preempted reportorial attention. Indeed, the large political events that summer had kept reportage down before as well as after Legionnaire's Disease. This is particularly noticeable in the TV coverage of the insurance struggle and its sudden outcome. On their evening news shows NBC gave rather more attention than did CBS, perhaps for reasons running back to differences of emphasis in March. A non-political program, technically respectable, caught in a tussle between President and Congress may have more intrinsic interest to editors or producers than one thought to be politicized and rotten to the core. The coverage on those networks lends this speculation credence. At any rate there was a rather dry spell in July and then, after the early August flurry, still another. This was a boon for CDC. Had investigative reporters had time heavy on their hands that summer—as for instance the next summer—swine flu could have been a gold mine whichever way one's predilections ran, non-political, rotten, or both.

Even so, the cumulative coverage of swine flu by all media,

from February through the early August scare and legislation, produced an extraordinary result. The Gallup Poll reported August 31 that 93 percent of all Americans had heard about the swine flu program; 53 percent intended to get shots. This bore out a separate poll commissioned by CDC.

There, the 53 percent intention occasioned disappointment and some apprehension. Cooper, after all, had set their sights on 95 percent. Besides, flu season would soon start and Kilbourne's expectation had still to be tested. In the absence of pandemic, they'd have done better to concern themselves about the challenge of that vast public awareness. It exposed them where their August flaps and fumbles showed them weak, on the external side of management, anticipating and adjusting to the public aspects. This was their blind side, as events would shortly emphasize again.

On October 1, mass immunization started in the states that had vaccine; from week to week others joined in. After three changes of plan since June, some states were prepared to move fast while others were almost inactive. Still, in the first 10 days over a million Americans got shots. These were all adults, of course; the new set of field trials was still under way; children were still in abeyance.

On October 11, in Pittsburgh, Pennsylvania, three persons over 70, all with cardiac conditions, dropped dead shortly after receiving swine flu shots at the same clinic. An alert UPI reporter picked up the story from a local paper and sent it over the wires; subsequent stories featured the fact that the same batch of Parke-Davis vaccine was involved. Pittsburgh is close to TV network news bureaus. Mini-cameras and crews were soon on their way. On October 12, the Allegheny County Coroner, Dr. Cyril Wecht, stepped forward to meet them. He told CBS:

> I think that . . . [a bad batch] of vaccine is definitely one possibility that must be considered. And that is why we want to see the [Federal] people here. . . .

Thereupon, the Allegheny County Health Department suspended flu shots. Nine states followed at once: Alaska, Illinois, Louisiana, Maine, New Mexico, Texas, Vermont, Virginia and Wisconsin. The wire service began a national body count.

That evening, Sencer held a press conference and offered calming words:

We have no evidence that there's anything wrong with the vaccine, but to be perfectly sure, the vaccine that is still in the field is being brought in for re-examination in Bethesda by the Bureau of Biologics. We are setting up a program to look into this in great depth, to reassure everyone that this is not a problem due to the vaccine, but just some of the inherent problems of providing preventative services to large numbers of people, particularly those who are elderly and have other underlying health problems.[20]

Wecht, the coroner, was not so easily put off. On October 13, he gave the autopsy results on two of his three corpses, heart failure, but hinted at negligence, not coincidence.

We know that substances injected into the vascular system directly produce a more exaggerated and certainly a more rapid reaction than when those same substances are injected into the body fat or muscle mass.[21]

Millar at CDC leaped to the defense of coincidence, and offered up some figures he might better have provided in advance.

We estimate . . . that among people 70-to-74-years of age something on the order of 10 to 12 deaths per 100,000 such people will occur every day. . . . We are seeing people who are dying within a day or so after vaccination. We expected to see that.[22]

CDC itself got into body-counting, and Millar competed with the wire services. For a while the number 33 was favored, later 41 on CDC's last count of Americans who had received flu shots and died of other causes. Meanwhile, for three straight days, swine flu was a big story on the network news, and safety questions were not left to eager coroners alone. The NBC Evening News of October 13 had Carole Simpson quoting a scientist recently identified in public with these matters: ". . . it's not safe."[23]

On October 14, the hullabaloo subsided. Ford and his family got televised flu shots. Cooper gave the press both lab reports establishing the vaccine's innocence and tough talk about "body count mentality." Allegheny County and five states announced resumption of inoculations; the other four said they would do so shortly. And, to top it all off, Walter Cronkite almost apologized. On his network radio broadcast he commented:

The qualifiers [in a "catastrophe" story like this one] never quite seem to repair the damage done by the initial statement. Many people are left with the distinct impression that the vaccine may be fatal. Health officials can talk until they are blue in the face but they so far have not been able to dispel that impression. . . .

The scare was set off when Pittsburgh halted its immunization program while the deaths of three elderly persons were investigated. All three had been immunized at the same clinic. No connection was found but the word was out. The repetition of stories which appeared to link death and vaccination have spread that damage like wildfire. Hopefully it will all die down but it will take considerable public relations efforts such as the President's well-publicized vaccination today.[24]

This gave inordinate satisfaction for the moment to the Coopers, Meriwethers, Sencers and Millars, which is too bad. In our view they didn't deserve it.

For we think that the whole episode was perfectly predictable: the coincident deaths in some city, the wire services, the nearby mini-cameras, the eager coroner (or Mayor or what-have-you), the human interest, hence the body count, and so forth. We think, therefore, that Federal sponsors of the program should have predicted it, briefed the states about it, passed the word to medical practitioners, alerted health officials in all major cities, and sat down with network news bureaus and wire service bureaus, all handy at Atlanta, seeking counsel. In the prevailing climate of press pride and touchiness, counsel might have been refused, which is no reason not to ask.

Cooper at the time expressed somewhat these sentiments. On October 14, James McManus reported on CBS News:

Dr. Cooper said he now wishes he had earlier and more strongly outlined possible events surrounding the program including deaths that might appear to be associated with the shots.[25]

So far as we can find, nothing of the sort was tried. "Temporally related deaths" were certainly anticipated in Hattwick's surveillance center. We understand that they had been discussed from time to time at higher levels. The problem loomed, but that was all; planning was discounted on the grounds that information spreads, and to alert the public might reduce the numbers willing to be immunized.

However that may be, alerting the public in an *un*planned way probably did reduce those numbers. It also emphasized some troubling undercurrents: whom would the program kill? old or young? poor or rich? black or white? All fall, ghetto acceptance rates were lower than suburban rates, for reasons obvious enough once stated, but again not worked through in advance. Although conscious of the problems of race and class, PHS and CDC made little impact on them—nor did they make provision for the public consequences of that failure.

From mid-October on, polls showed a downward drift of persons who intended to be immunized. Absolute numbers of those actually inoculated rose for a while as state plans took hold. During "Pittsburgh week" and despite it, 2.4 million people were immunized. A month later those numbers rose to 6.4 million for the second week of November. A month after that, however, they had dropped back to 2.3 million for the second week of December.

By then a number of factors other than fear were working to cut numbers. In November the children's dosage question was resolved precisely as had been foreseen in June: children should receive two doses of the split vaccine, but there was only enough of it to immunize one child in every dozen. Moreover, there was little participation from private physicians. They accounted, all told, for only 15 percent of inoculations, and were anything but vocal in support of immunization. Our unscientific sample suggests that many were indifferent, others confused, and most disgruntled: "Politics." Kilbourne had urged on Sencer weekly bulletins to every private doctor. Had Kilbourne's expected pandemic come to pass this would have been essential. But CDC had acted on the expectation, not the suggestion. Private physicians were, above all, uninformed.

And then, of course, there was no swine flu, or almost none.

One case, not directly traceable to pigs, showed up in Concordia, Missouri. That was all. Millions came down with other respiratory ailments passed from human to human that fall. But with this one exception there were none the swine flu virus could have caused, or vaccine cured.

Between October 1 and December 16, more than 40 million Americans received swine flu shots through Sencer's program. (Defense and VA programs accounted for some millions more.) This is twice the number ever immunized before for any influenza virus in a single season. Considering the obstacles it is an impressive number. It also is a number oddly distributed. Some states, albeit small ones, inoculated 80 percent of their adults in that time period. Others immunized not more than 10 percent. Delaware was at the top of that range, New York City near the bottom. Variations in between are striking: Houston, Texas, inoculated only 10 percent of its adults, while San Antonio, Texas, immunized nearly one-third. Despite coincident deaths, Pittsburgh, Pennsylvania, vaccinated nearly 43 percent while Philadephia, home of Legionnaire's Disease, managed but 23 percent. And so forth.[26] These variations cry out for explanation. So far as we know CDC has not pursued them and may lack the resources to do so. HEW would gain if Congress asked the GAO to do it.

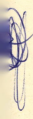

We suggest a study by the GAO because our own informal sampling poses puzzles about what may actually have happened. We are wary of the future capabilities at state and local levels. We fear that Federal programs may be hollow shells. What we now think occurred, on insufficient evidence, is that Federal officials tried to influence state counterparts and they in turn tried variably to energize their local health departments. The locals, not the others, were decisive for most states. In each city and county, four things may have come together to determine performance: First was the availability of vaccine and consent forms, matters of complaint (along with children's dosages). Second was the underlying attitude of residents, welcoming or fearing mass immunization. Third was competence, indicated we think by relative success with immunization programs already in place. And fourth was conviction on the part of somebody at once willing and able to take local leadership.

Believers in the threat of a pandemic did far more than non-believers. The counties of this country certainly were split between the two. And what divided them may rest on nothing more than faith, hunch or contacts.

We do not suggest that strategies and planning, locally or statewide, made no difference to the variations in performance. But as of now we have no judgment on the point. Only a detailed investigation at both local and state levels can decide.

One state that was conscientious in its conduct of the national program was Minnesota, where nearly two-thirds of the eligible adults were immunized. In the third week of November, a physician there reported to his local health authorities a patient who had contracted an ascending paralysis, called Guillain-Barré syndrome, following immunization. The physician said he had just learned of this possible side effect from a cassette-tape discussion of flu vaccination prepared for the continuing education of family practitioners by a California specialist. The Minnesota immunization program officer, Denton R. Peterson, dutifully called CDC and spoke to one of the surveillance physicians there. The latter expressed no interest in this single case, but Peterson was sufficiently bothered to conduct a literature search and did indeed discover previous case reports. "We felt we were sitting on a bomb," he told us. Within a week three more cases, one fatal, were reported to Peterson. Two came from a single neurologist who remarked that he had observed this complication of flu vaccine during his residency training. More anxious than ever, Peterson again called CDC, where the surveillance center was just being told by phone of three more cases in Alabama. The next day they learned of an additional case in New Jersey. By then CDC was taking the problem seriously. Center staff surveyed neurologists in eleven states to ascertain the relative risk of this rare disease (estimated at 5000 cases annually) among vaccinated and unvaccinated. When the preliminary results suggested an increased risk among the vaccinated, Sencer sought advice from usual sources: NIAID, BoB, ACIP and his own people. The statistical association did not convince them all.

But what struck everybody, sensitized by their long summer, was the thought: until the risk (if any) is established, it cannot be put into a consent form! The statistical relationship would have to be reviewed and immunization halted in the interim. After everything that had already happened, everybody took that to mean virtual termination. Even the least imaginative could conjure up the television shots of victims in their beds, wheel chairs, and respirators.

With some trepidation about White House willingness to stop, Sencer called Cooper on December 16, and fortuitously reached him in the White House Staff Mess, lunching with Cavanaugh. Mathews by chance was at another table. The three huddled quickly; Cooper then excused himself and made a call to Salk. The switchboard reached Salk in Paris. Without enthusiasm he concurred in Sencer's view. Cooper and the others then walked down the hall to Ford. He heard them out, sighed and agreed. For most intents and purposes the swine flu program was over. With no disease in sight nine months after Ford's announcement, even a rare side effect could turn him around.

That afternoon Cooper announced suspension of the swine flu program, saying that he was acting "in the interest of safety of the public, in the interest of credibility, and in the interest of the practice of good medicine."[27]

Press comments were not kind. The TV anchormen conveyed no sense of loss. And five days later Harry Schwartz contributed an Op Ed piece in the *New York Times*. Entitled "Swine Flu Fiasco," it rounded off the points that he had previously made in anonymity:

The sorry debacle of the swine flu vaccine program provides a fitting end point to the misunderstandings and misconceptions that have marked Government approaches to health care during the last eight years. . . .

Any reasonable effort to assign responsibility for this state of affairs must call attention to at least the following elements:

(1) The scarcity in the White House and in Congress of officials with sufficient sophistication in medical problems to be able to put biological reality before political expediency. . . .

(2) The excessive confidence of the Government medical bureaucracy and its outside experts in urging the vaccination program

on the country while playing down the uncertainties arising from the fact that medical science still knows comparatively little about the origin and spread of influenza epidemics. . . .

(3) The self-interest of Government health bureaucracy which saw in the swine flu threat the ideal chance to impress the nation with the capabilities of saving money and lives by preventing disease.

In our view his first element overplays the politics. For the rest we offer a refinement. The "heavies" here were seven or eight personal agendas which happened to converge in the remembered light of 1918.

10

CALIFANO COMES IN

The swine flu program had not been much of an issue in the 1976 campaign. Jimmy Carter had disdained a flu shot just at the time Ford was receiving his. But this was in the ninth month after Fort Dix and without a case in sight: political marginalia.

Still, for many Democrats attentive to health issues, the program had bit deeper. It had served to symbolize what they regarded as a cumulative record of deception and ineptitude on the Republican side. This evidently was the attitude of Joseph Califano, a Washington attorney who had headed President Johnson's White House staff for domestic affairs. Given to working long hours, Califano rarely saw the television news but regularly read the *New York Times*, and he knew many journalists and congressmen who shared the perspective of Harry Schwartz. When Carter named Califano Secretary-designate of HEW, that perspective played a part in his approach to his new duties.

The first duty was to bring in a new team. Califano set out to clean house in health. This almost automatically ruled Cooper out of office, on grounds of symbolism independent of his record, and regardless of support for him developing in Congress and in Carter's entourage. Determined to be his own man on appointments, Califano set up his own talent search. By January 20, 1977, this had not produced a replacement for Cooper, in part because reorganization was envisaged, and Dickson became Acting Assistant Secretary. Dr. Donald Fredrickson was staying on as head of NIH, which seemed to show that a clean house need not be clean-swept.

Sencer's future was decided at the end of January after a canvass of external views. On balance it was felt that he had headed CDC too long, over ten years, that swine flu had diminished his effectiveness, and that now was a better time than most to make the change. On February 4, Hale Champion, the Undersecretary, called Sencer to Washington for a discussion of his future, told him he would be replaced in due course, offered him time to decide his next steps, and promised confidentiality. (Champion spoke under some constraint, aware that formally the Surgeon General, not the Secretary, named directors of CDC.) Sencer said he wanted to discuss the matter with a few associates and warned that HEW leaked like a sieve. They parted amicably; in retrospect each wonders if the other fully grasped what he was trying to convey.

By February 4 Califano, two weeks in office, was facing his first swine flu decision; whether or not to release bivalent vaccine.

The program's suspension, December 16, had been less definitive than press obituaries made it seem. It had been for the stated purpose of examining the link between inoculation and Guillain-Barré. Hattwick's surveillance center produced data and the ACIP reviewed it first on December 29, 1976, and again on January 14, 1977. The risk of developing Guillain-Barré syndrome seemed to be eleven times greater with vaccination than without. But the risk was still remote, about 1 in 105,000, and the risk of death but 1 in 2 million.

On January 14, the ACIP recommended limited resumption of the swine flu program so that the Victoria vaccine locked up in bivalent doses could be made available again to high-risk groups. Sencer promptly sent this on to Cooper, who responded with questions. These Sencer pursued in a telephone poll of the states. Almost all said they would make bivalent vaccine readily available for high-risk groups, two-thirds said they also would make monovalent available; only a few were prepared to consider resuming an active public campaign. Short of a campaign, the estimated cost of restarting the program was only $15–30,000, the cost of printing new consent forms.

On January 17 Sencer reported back. Cooper now expressed his personal agreement but refused to act. The new Administration was but three days off; leave it to them. There was no hurry. Swine flu was epidemic nowhere in the world, Victoria nowhere in America.

Twelve days later, Victoria flu erupted in a nursing home in Miami, Florida. Califano now faced the decision Cooper had put off. There was no one else to face it. Improvising as he went, advised mainly by Fredrickson and Dr. David Hamburg, head of the Institute of Medicine, the Secretary settled on a straightforward procedure. First, Sencer's recommendation and the work behind it would be set before an *ad hoc* advisory group of broader character and less commitment than the ACIP, and with prestigious chairmen from outside the flu establishment. The deliberations of the group would be both covered by the press and open to the public (which in Washington means organizations) and there would be time for comment from the audience. Califano would appear himself and hear as much as he could. Then, the group would draw conclusions and present them to him for his own decision.

While Fredrickson and Hamburg put together the group's membership, Califano wrote Carter, apprised him of the problem, and explained the procedure. Members of the old ACIP would be included.

But in light of the controversy surrounding the immunization program, I will ask other experts to join the special advisory group so that we will have as broad and objective a base as possible under the circumstances. The group will be led by two of our nation's most distinguished scientists, Dr. John Knowles and Dr. Ivan Bennett.[28]

Knowles was President of the Rockefeller Foundation and Bennett the Dean of New York University Medical Center. Califano had recruited them himself.

Thus the White House was at once informed and kept away. This was not to be a presidential decision. The new President was evidently satisfied. As for the new staff, they and Califano had divergent views on many things, but not on this.

Califano's special group met Monday, February 7, for an all-day session in the conference room on the 8th floor of HEW's new headquarters, since named for Hubert Humphrey. When the conferees arrived they found one feature Califano had not intended, television coverage. Fearing lest it distract advisers and detract from the discussions, he had ruled it out. ABC, the network pool, failed to get the word and had set up the room before the HEW press people noticed. Assistant Secretary Eileen Shanahan then sensibly let everything alone. Advisers seemed not to be much distracted, discussion proceeded, and Califano had a new element in his procedure.

There was only one unhappy consequence of television coverage, this not attributable to its paraphernalia but to insufficient planning in the Secretary's entourage. During the morning meeting which Califano attended, Ben Heineman, his Executive Assistant, got word that Sencer's departure was being carried on one of the wire services. Sencer, of course, was also at the meeting, shepherding his people, making the presentation. Fearing that Califano might get a direct question from attending press, and in the circumstances issue a denial without knowing what was on the ticker, Heineman sent word to him about it. Califano then called Sencer aside and standing along the wall they talked for some time, out of earshot but in view of all. The press was now on to the story, so much so that at noon a one-line announcement was made by HEW. In mid-afternoon a wire service reporter finally cornered Sencer; he elaborated off-the-record.

At the end of the day, with reporters pressing both of them, Califano held an impromptu press conference. After complimenting Sencer for distinguished service, he said he wanted a director of his "own choosing. . . . Sencer's been at CDC for 16 years and director for 10 years. I think it's important that institutions be rejuvenated and revitalized."[29] The universal assumption of his auditors and of the network commentators on that night's new shows was that the deed had been done on the spot, up against the wall, to make plain Califano's distance from, and dislike for, the swine flu program: Sencer the human sacrifice. In professional circles this won him deserved sympathy. The CDC-ers present were appalled, their colleagues in Atlanta still more so. This, it seemed to many, was the government's reward for a career in public health and for devotion to their agency. Thus Califano's reputation there began.

As a leading epidemiologist remarked to us:

Sencer was canned for doing his job; it shows you Califano is nothing but a politician. . . . He thinks he's a smart lawyer, but he doesn't know the first thing about health.

Three months later, Califano somewhat cooled the CDC reaction by choosing from inside Sencer's assistant director, Foege, as the new head of the agency. Foege had not been long at Atlanta. He had come there following his own signal success in the smallpox eradication program. His ego thus was independent of the agency. Moreover, unlike Sencer, or Cooper for that matter, Foege was known for ego control.

Aside from the Sencer problem, Califano's improvised procedure, television included, was a great success with most of those attending and for HEW. At the day's end the advisory group recommended to the Secretary that suspension of the bivalent vaccine be lifted for the sake of high-risk groups facing Victoria flu outbreaks. With no swine flu outbreaks, the monovalent vaccine should continue in suspense.

The next day the Secretary announced his acceptance of those recommendations. One of the things he had sought from his procedure was an opportunity to tell the press: "Everything I heard, you heard if you sat through the meeting." Now he could do just that, and did. He could also say to interest groups and critics of every sort: "You had a right to be heard, and a *chance*; nothing was done behind your back." After the swine flu program, Califano thought these things great assets, and still does, elements in building (and rebuilding) credibility. Media reaction to his limited resumption strengthened that belief. Harry Schwartz wrote still another editorial for the *New York Times*: ". . . The Government stands now where it should have stood all along: focused on high-risk individuals and poised to do more, but only if necessary."[30]

The *Washington Post* editorialized:

> It was not an easy decision to make, given all the unknowns and unknowables involved, and it strikes us as a sensible one that carefully balanced all the risks involved. But what struck us almost as forcefully was the wide-open way that it was made—the "sunshine" approach, if you will.[31]

We have heard but one caveat, procedural, not substantive. Stallones, who had flown up from Texas for the meeting, found the conference room repellent—cold decor with chilly temperature—and fellow panelists excessively Eastern: New York–Boston almost all. He commented to us:

> I am not very enamored of the Eastern establishment, nor do I much enjoy being practically alone in it. . . . Surely they could try harder on that dimension.

Surely they can, but not perhaps a Fredrickson or a Hamburg in an hour's time.

The improvised procedure of February 7 worked so well that a month later, when it came time to review ACIP recommendations for the 1977–78 flu season, a comparable *ad hoc* group at Califano's level was again laid on; he again received its views, again he took them as his own. Not surprisingly, the recommendations were conservative as first proposed from CDC and as approved by him: private manufacture of Victoria vaccine for high-risk groups. Here was a complete reversion to 1975, no Federal programming at all. Despite an unexpected epidemic of the Texas strain (akin to the Victoria), this outcome was as well received in public as the last and carried Federal policy along until the news of Russian flu late in 1977.

With these two *ad hoc* performances in February and March, Califano put a period to the swine flu program. What remained were doses in the refrigerator, consent forms on the shelf, and policy issues he had not yet addressed.

11

LEGACIES

The swine flu program ended, but in terms of Federal policy it left at least three legacies. With these the Secretary still is dealing or has yet to deal. One is a national commission on immunization policy. Another is liability policy. The third is an expanded Federal role in influenza immunization. The three interlock. They still evolve. They carry far beyond March 1977, the month we made our stopping-point for detailed reconstruction. But during 1977, while we worked on 1976, we tried to keep an eye on these three legacies. We offer a comment on each.

A National Commission

The idea of a commission on immunization policy is indistinguishable from the history of the two National Immunization Conferences, in November 1976 and in April 1977, which Cooper planned as the fulfillment of a pledge to Senator Kennedy. The pledge had been extracted during hearings in September 1976, after the tort claims statute had been followed by delivery delays. Kennedy seemed eager for a long-lasting body to review and pull together every aspect of the issues that had plagued the swine flu program.

. . . I do not really feel that a conference is sufficient to deal with the kind of problems we have here, the problems we are really concerned with and talking about and which are raised in this issue [availability of vaccine] here.

I think a conference can be useful under certain circumstances. . . . I think all of us who attend them do obtain some degree of information or knowledge; but due to the kind of indepth work that I think needs to be done, . . . I think it needs a commission.

. . .

We are really going to insist on this.[32]

He settled for the promise of two conferences.

Cooper organized the first one as a sounding board for those who felt the swine flu program to have been at once desirable and problematical, problematic because unprecedented, hence underprepared. The whole influenza cast of characters turned out and more besides: CDC and NIAID and BoB staffs, with advisers, public health professionals, pediatricians, laboratory chiefs and some executives from the drug companies, epidemiologists from state health departments, even the likes of Leslie Cheek, and better still, insurance company vice presidents, together with a scattering from voluntary agencies, public interest groups, congressional staffs, and press. After discussion, the Conference divided into six work groups which were asked to report four months hence at a second conference. These groups covered a lot of ground: Production, R & D, Consent, Liability, Public Awareness, and Policy. Their reports were duly printed and distributed three weeks before the second conference. At that affair, the same people, more or less, assembled again, discussed again, and adjourned, leaving the reports to work their way to agency or congressional action.

Cooper was ten weeks gone by the time of the April Conference, but Califano showed up full of expressed interest. This gained immediate approval followed by drawn-out disappointment. Califano's staff work at the time had not sufficed to count the cost of his expressiveness. He had already announced his immunization initiatives for children, incidentally over-promis-

ing in Cooper's wake. Now he went to this affair to demonstrate
how much the general subject mattered to him and how differently he felt about such departmental doings than had Mathews,
the phantom. But soon enough, staff found they disagreed with
many portions of those working group reports. Califano was
more than willing to hold still. At lower levels this appeared
erratic.

Three of the six reports had featured a proposal eagerly accepted by most conferees, a National Immunization Commission or Policy Council. This was an adaptation of the Kennedy
idea. Its authors meant to substitute for both the old ACIP and
Califano-like *ad hoc*-ery a permanent body at the apex of
decision-making:

The commission should have the responsibility for reviewing and
advising the Secretary on all matters concerning immunization policies, priorities, and practices as they may affect the public health of
the United States. . . . continuing awareness of the effectiveness,
safety, need for the availability of existing . . . and additional
vaccines. . . . stimulation and support of . . . research . . . training
of personnel . . . public and professional education. . . . judgment of
the need for public vaccination campaigns; review of the present
system of vaccine administration, both public and private; and provision of long range support of programs to assure adequate immunization levels of the population. . . .[33]

Many persons had combined to produce this proposal. Among
them was Salk, for reasons running back to his original agenda
of a year before. His interest was well known to Kennedy
through Dr. Lawrence Horowitz, a subcommittee staffer. And
the work groups that proposed it represented other interests too,
ranging from the professors, researchers, and consumers who
might sit on it to the three agencies whose stabilized relationships had barely been defense enough against recent upheavals:
CDC, BoB and NIAID. A National Commission could be
counted on to spread stability one and two levels up, easing
the way for them.

Two difficulties strike us but were not voiced at the conference and perhaps struck no one there. One difficulty is that
along with stability a body of this sort would also bring, in time,
its members' own agendas and their mutual accommodations,

turning into but another agency among the many predisposed in given ways. Its predispositions almost surely would include a growing role for federal immunization. They also almost surely would reflect the preferences of staff, and staffers more than likely would be drawn from the three agencies below: CDC, BoB and NIAID. Even if the higher-level body had a wholly separate staff, it could not help but seek to bargain with those three for positions they could advocate together.

To lose *ad hoc*-ery for that strikes us as a poor bargain.

Moreover, such a body would, we think, be bound in time to fall into the orbit of the congressional subcommittees. Ultimately, Kennedy and Rogers with their staffs would be better able than a transient Secretary to affect the course of "national immunization policy." Whether this is good or bad depends on where one sits.

In a June conversation with his then special assistant, Dr. Michael McGinnis (now a Deputy Assistant Secretary for Health), Secretary Califano indicated his preference for dispensing with a commission or council. His reasons were his own, not ours. In ordinary times he saw it duplicating work that PHS executives and their advisers, or his office, ought to do. Should an emergency like swine flu arise, he might turn to his recently created Ethics Advisory Board. The Board was chaired by James Gaither, a San Francisco lawyer and a former aide in Califano's White House years. If special talents were required they could find them as before, *ad hoc*.

In our opinion there is nothing wrong with this, except that Messrs. Kennedy and Horowitz may not have got a national commission off their minds. Salk has not, as he told us in December 1977. The second-level bureaucrats assuredly have not. They raise it still at any opportunity. And various consumer groups still have it on their lists, joined happily by the Pharmaceutical Manufacturers Association eager for alliances across the market.

Liability Legislation

The liability problem remains at the heart of immunization policy so long as manufacturers and their insurers insist on special treatment for Federally sponsored programs. Either such programs are circumscribed, if not ruled out, or duty to warn and legal costs are federalized. As Dull had done in 1976 and others earlier, the National Immunization Conference and its work group on the subject naturally put immunization first: to preserve options and facilitate development of Federal programs, the private sector *ought* to have its way. Whether this meant tort claims procedure as with swine flu, or indemnification, or some way of compensating victims, was subsidiary. The sooner a choice was made, and legislation passed, the better for immunization.

That there is an array of other issues, quite apart from immunization, issues of precedent, of equity, of cost, of public-private balance, of administrative and judicial roles, has never impressed persons who put immunizing first.

In 1977, the new hands at HEW were in no hurry to dig into this one. Childhood immunization, they found, could be pursued by contractual assumption of the duty to warn, provided that the states assumed it, rather than HEW, even though the vaccines were procured with Federal dollars. The manufacturers and their insurers went along with that. It eased their fears of baseless suits. The states, they felt, would rouse less public ire and state laws in many places would discourage suits in general. Best of all, the childhood programs were small-scale compared to swine flu.

Califano thus was able to pursue immediate concerns through spring and summer without facing the hard issues embedded in long-term solutions.

The tort claims legislation of the year before had mandated from HEW a report on alternatives after its expiration. This had been a Rogers interest. The report was expected by his subcommittee. Mindful of that, Cooper had set up in PHS an interagency committee, chaired by Dr. James Cooper, with representation from OGC. When the new regime came in, Cooper proceeded more or less alone. His office served as a convenient place to send the liability report from April's Immunization Conference. Through the next months, Califano's staff and OGC alike assumed that somehow James Cooper was coping. He wasn't. In late July his draft report from the Secretary to Congress reached Rick Cotton of the HEW Executive Secretariat. Cotton considered it unsatisfactory. He sounded an alarm and forced a search for substitutes, turning, among others, to McGinnis and to Richard Beattie, Barrett's successor as Deputy General Counsel.

McGinnis thereupon took up the task of getting a respectable report prepared, and pulled together a scratch team to do it. He seized the incoming White House Fellow, Dr. Louise Liang, and he talked one of Beattie's newest lawyers, Linda Donaldson, into "part-time" commitment. Beattie was resistant. Donaldson had been recruited as a general-purpose aide to help with matters of immediate concern to Califano. As Beattie put it to us:

I told her not to let herself get sucked into anything. But she did. I was concerned about her. She was new; it was a new issue to her. And we needed her on other things. I felt that the laboring oar in drafting the report should have been carried by Health. Given Joe's own demands on us we were trying to run a special "law firm for the Secretary," and we only had about six lawyers free for the work. She was supposed to be one of them. . . .

To give the Donaldson-Liang team time, HEW twice asked for extensions of the statutory deadline. Substantively it was worth it. In little more than three months they, with Beattie's help, produced the first thoroughgoing brief on liability, assessing issues and detailing options, that HEW had ever had. In March 1976, it would have been an invaluable guide. In November 1977, Califano felt no need to act precipitously and he had incentives not to. The precedential effects of all alternatives were sobering. The issues were complex. Besides, the Donaldson report led logically toward compensation for the victim of immunization, removing redress from judicial to administrative process. At Justice, the Neil Petersons were sure to snicker: "Uncle Joe and the do-gooders." Califano's instincts pulled both ways. He thus forbore to make a rapid choice among alternatives, agreeing to give Congress in November only an analysis without recommendations. In his words to us:

The issues underlying . . . are very tough. . . . We still haven't enough information on some things. . . . The decisions will be tough. I need time to soak before I make them and take a stand. I know I'll have to do that but I certainly don't want to do it in a rush if I don't have to . . . and I don't unless we have another drastic antigenic shift, or if more manufacturers get out of the business, so we're down to one who's thinking about quitting, something like that.

We think the point well made. But CDC-ers, NIAID-ers and the like have never heard it. The immunologists have frequently found Califano baffling (irritating, infuriating), never more than on this issue. To them he is no phantom, but instead a sort of cross between the "arbitrary" Tzar and the "impenetrable" sphinx.

There the matter rested at the turn of 1978, waiting on events.

A New Immunization Initiative

The reports of the Immunization Conference had implied an enlarged Federal role in influenza immunization, not on the swine flu scale, except perhaps in an emergency, but larger than before. What was now suggested was Federal money for vaccine and technical assistance in its distribution. At Millar's level in CDC there was a lot of interest (if not active promotion).

CDC lives by a web of intricate relationships between its human cadres of epidemiologists and public health advisers, and the money it dispenses to the states for special projects. Here, in sight, was a new project grant.

But nothing came of those conference reports. They were released in March 1977. The new Assistant Secretary, Dr. Julius Richmond, did not even take office until four months later. Califano showed no independent interest. McGinnis sat on them.

In the fall of 1977, the concerned CDC-ers took a new tack—pandemic planning. They joined counterparts in NIAID and BoB to urge on Richmond's deputy, Dr. Joyce Lashof, a working group to think about the coming of the antigenic shift which swine flu wasn't. When she agreed, they constituted themselves as such. And when her office asked for a report (a query probably inspired), they drafted one proposing Federally supported immunization every year for high-risk groups as the essential feature of pandemic planning. Generously defined and conscientiously pursued, this could bring a quarter of the population annually within the purview of routine delivery systems. With those systems oiled and ready, their expansion to meet a severe pandemic, even another 1918, should be simpler, more predictable and surer than the improvised and often altered distribution schemes of 1976. Meanwhile CDC itself could weave a stronger web. And influenza immunization would be on the map among established Federal programs, ready for emergency enlargement.

This argument was in draft form by mid-November 1977. Note that it rested on a chilling afterview, not previously expressed by CDC, of limited state capabilities in 1976. And the capacity of states to learn by doing was asserted, not assessed. That a delivery system for 200 million could expand from 50 million better than from nothing may not be as plain a proposition as it seems. At one extreme is Sabin arguing that nationwide immunization in good time could only be accomplished through locally organized volunteer brigades, prepared in advance. At the opposite extreme is Rockefeller evidently thinking that a dangerous pandemic calls for federalization, or resort to the armed forces. With no close analysis of capabilities, pandemic planning assumed state-run programs.

Planning was overtaken at the end of 1977 by the prospect of a new pandemic from the Russian flu foreseen for 1978. That form of influenza, exactly like a mild virus last seen in the mid-fifties, had spread from east to west across the Soviet Union and seemed about to spread to Western Europe and America. The prospect was explored in successive *ad hoc* meetings, each open to the press with the third televised: the first in Atlanta, the second in Bethesda, and the third in Califano's conference room. This was *ad hoc*-ery carried to an extreme, but that is a matter of taste. Under Califano, public meetings become status symbols. By the time of the third meeting, January 30, 1978, an inspection team had returned from the Soviet Union and Russian flu had reached the United States. This facilitated a consensus on the likelihood of further outbreaks in this country all during 1978 and into 1979. Russian flu would be competing with and might replace the current strains of Texas and Victoria flu.

Part of the consensus, as reported to the Secretary, was a Federal program funding state procurement for some 30 million doses of trivalent vaccine. This could assure that Russian vaccine (combined with others marketed in 1977) would be available for use in high-risk groups.[34] If the *states* placed the orders, spokesmen for the manufacturers had said they would fill them without Federal liability legislation, provided the states assumed duty to warn. The states, it was thought, would attract fewer suits. There thus was no Federal procurement. But there would be Federal funding and some technical assistance in the form of a new project grant.

This program, not coincidentally, was a version of pandemic planning tailored to the worsened flu prospects for 1978. The justification became deaths attributed to influenza, focusing attention on the high-risk groups. If good for 1978 this would be good in any year, since influenza was a source of deaths in every year. The program contemplated adaptation, year by year, to meet anticipated drifts and shifts of the flu virus. In the present state of knowledge, anticipations could be wrong, there was no help for that. But public understanding might be strengthened in the process and state capabilities as well. If planning for a bad year was not emphasized, neither was it forgotten. As one public health official said to us:

It will take maybe 25 years to get this right, to be wise in the spring about what's going to happen in the fall, but meanwhile lives will certainly be saved, everybody will be gaining valuable experience, and the public will get quite an education on influenza.

So Califano was told January 30. Behind the consensus of his public meeting there lay staff work and advocacy by the erstwhile pandemic planners. Foege, not a rash man, had already sounded out congressional aides, citing costs of $15–20 million. The Secretary, in response, questioned the willingness of states to take the funds, procure the vaccine and distribute it, while contracting to warn. A CDC round-up by phone showed two-thirds aquiescent, others possible. Califano also questioned definition of "high-risk." He acknowledged those of any age with "chronic medical conditions"—mainly cardiac and respiratory illnesses—and everybody over 65. Age 65 was the conventional base for recognizing a statistical relationship between aging and death from influenza. The relationship starts to show at 50 and the pandemic planners would have liked to label all above that age "high-risk." But after pressing senior PHS advisers, Califano got agreement on the higher base. This reduced from 66 to 42 million people those whom HEW defined as at high risk. Of these it expected 20 percent to be reached by existing services, and hoped that Federal grants could bring that up to 40 percent in one year's time, to 60 percent later. These targets translated into dollar costs of $15 million for the first year, $20 million for the second and unspecified amounts thereafter.

Satisfied with this, Califano did not try to find the funds internally. Dollar tradeoff offends doctors. He didn't like it either. Instead, on February 16, he sent his people to the OMB for a supplemental appropriation. The Administration had changed, but not the government: Zafra, still suspicious, was waiting to receive them. This time Zafra had available to him, alongside OMB in the Executive Office of the President, the Science Adviser's Office (formally the Office of Science and Technology Policy, OSTP), with an assistant director in health-related matters. The latter strengthened Zafra's hand and sharpened budget questions, urging, among other things, that healthy people over 65 need not invariably be presumed high risks.

The OMB examiners thereupon recommended a still smaller program, and they wanted it absorbed without additional appropriations. The issue reached the Budget Director and Califano compromised (on paper). He got a program of his size but funded separately for only its first year; the second year costs were to be absorbed by PHS. This was agreed, Congress willing. OMB examiners assumed that Congress would be only too willing to undo the absorption scheme (tradeoffs in public health were no more usual at the top of Capitol Hill than at the bottom). Thereupon the President included $15 million for the first year in a supplemental appropriation request. It went to Congress February 23, 1978.

At the same time, with OMB clearance HEW asked Congress for a permanent authorization. This invoked the Kennedy and Rogers subcommittees. Their response turned out to be more problematical than the Administration had foreseen. The Rogers subcommittee was insistent on receiving first a version of the liability report for which it had been waiting since the previous September. The Kennedy subcommittee had some members scoffing at a program ". . . from the same folks who brought us swine flu." As we write, neither subcommittee has produced a bill; appropriations are remote without one.

Still, two years after Sencer's action-memorandum Califano has endorsed a long-term version of the "minimum response" Sencer rejected then. If Congress acts, influenza will have joined rubella, measles, polio, among continuing, accepted, Federal immunization initiatives. This offers a perspective on the swine flu story. At the least it indicates what CDC has learned.

It also shows what influenza specialists have gained. If Congress does not act, the endorsement remains and flu is still a part of more agendas than before.

12

REFLECTIONS

So much for the swine flu story as we understand it now. The story conveys lessons large and small. Many of them leap out of the narrative. These we won't belabor. There is no need, for example, to suggest that Ford—or by extension Carter—should not have been out front. The thing suggests itself. But we *are* moved to offer further comment now on certain critical phenomena: program reviews, implementation analyses, media reactions, agency reputations and slippery diseases.

Mindful of our charge, these five bear on decision-making at the level of the HEW Secretary.

1. Building a Base for Program Review

In its notable report on the swine flu program, presented to Congress June 27, 1977, the General Accounting Office made one major recommendation:

. . . when decisions must be based on very limited scientific data, HEW should establish key points at which the program should be formally reevaluated.

With some justice, Sencer, among others, says that this is nothing new, indeed was done in 1976, except for the matter of form. There *were* three reevaluations of a sort, one in June after the first field trials, one in July, leading the President to push Congress, and the third in December, leading to suspension.

What more could anyone want? By way of answer, the GAO Report puts stress on form, on step-by-step review matching the steps in initial decision. December perhaps qualifies; June and July do not. We have no quarrel with this, but would go farther. As we see June and July, they demonstrate an aching need for something besides form.

The need is two-fold: first, a tracing out of the relationships between deadlines and each decision; second, an explicit statement of assumptions underlying each decision. As for deadlines, Sencer's action-memorandum of March 1976, with its two-week go-or-no-go, actually obscured, not clarified, relationships between deadlines and individual decisions. Arguably the decision to *begin* manufacturing (prepare recombinants and purchase eggs) was under such tight timing. But the decision to institute a mass immunization program was not. These could, and we believe should, have been separated at the outset.

Still, no distinctions among deadlines could have contributed to subsequent review without explicit analysis of the assumptions on which Sencer's all-rolled-into-one decision rested. Explicit means detail, not just strong possibility of a pandemic, risking another 1918, and an available technology, but also *high*-yield eggs, *one* dose per person, *high* efficacy, *unparalleled* acceptance, *favorable* publicity, *sustained* congressional support, *wide* private involvement, *adequate* state operations, *three* months to complete vaccinations, *no* useful stockpiling, *no* liability legislation, *few* (if any) opportunity costs, et cetera. In short, we advocate a comprehensive definition and review of assumptions everyone can see and weigh before decision and remember after. The review thus should be public. This seems to us a proper base for formal reevaluation.

Without it, we doubt reevaluators will be any better off than Ford was in July and early August 1976. Having publicly expressed in March no "ifs" except uncertainty about the coming of pandemic—which did not distinguish likelihoods in spring from those in summer, or differentiate spread from severity—he had no grounds to think about a change. As long as Cooper told him "it" remained a possibility with probability "unknown," Ford was stuck. Anyone would be.

We can see two ways to derive the details and distinctions for a useful analysis of the decision. One is to get the issue posed according to its component parts and argued in probabilistic terms. The other is to hunt for answers to the question Sencer once was asked by Alexander, in effect:

What evidence on which things, when and why, would make us change the course we now propose, and to what?

We do not see these two as mutually exclusive, and we think both are of use. Either would allow for reassessment of earlier decisions. The first may be best but will be hard indeed to get from public health officials. If so, the second becomes the Secretary's recourse. It is the nearest substitute we can suggest for probability analysis.

For purposes of sharpening assumptions and distinguishing them, nothing beats an exercise in probability. Deciding on a swine flu program is like placing a bet without knowing the odds. A serious stake in the outcome ought to concentrate the mind on breaking down the issue and scrounging for anything that might inform judgment. If one has "scientific" evidence from laboratory tests, one need not scrounge, but swine flu decisions are not like that. Expertise counts for a lot, but only by way of informing subjective judgment. To assign a number to the likelihood that something will occur is to expose one's judgment for comparison with that of others. This leads to explicitness about everyone's reasons. If two people assign different numbers, the question becomes, why? That starts them digging into the detail of their own—and each other's—reasoning.

But doctors, at least of the older generation, rarely think in terms of subjective probabilities and, if asked, dislike it. Some of the scientists involved with the swine flu decision did participate in an exercise to estimate the probabilities of an epidemic and its severity. This was not done as part of any decision-making deliberation, but as an academic exercise, a favor for a colleague writing a paper.[35] As scientists accustomed to thinking about experiments and "truth," they were uncomfortable expressing subjective estimates, even if based on expert knowledge and experience. They resented having to quantify their judgments.

Indeed, many think that it is unprofessional to express judgments in terms they cannot call scientific, worse still to express them in the presence of laymen. They see placing precise numbers on uncertainties as an incitement to public misunderstanding. Sencer and Cooper were proud of their refusal to put numbers on the possibility of a pandemic, proud to refuse Mathews, still more Ford. That augurs ill for any Secretary's persuasiveness in this regard with their successors.

Doctors, like other people, often think simplistically when, as so often happens, they must judge despite themselves on grounds other than laboratory evidence. Stallones explained to us that in his view the logic of decision at the ACIP meeting, March 10, 1976, is best conveyed by a simple, four-cell matrix. A program curbing a pandemic equals public health, ditto a program without a pandemic, ditto neither; only in the fourth cell, a pandemic without a program, does the public health suffer avoidable harm. And health was an absolute value. This is as simplistic as Sencer's next step, bundling up all pieces of the issue into one decision with one deadline, and pressing it on his Secretary. "Strong possibility with probability unknown," once down on paper, leakable at will, is at an opposite extreme from the detailed definition of relevant assumptions we suggest that the decision-maker seek.

But turning around tendencies like these is probably best done without demanding numbers which offend professional pride and inclination.

The question ACIP left unanswered is the next best source of the explicitness and detail we suggest: "Which evidence would make us alter course to what?" Meetings of expert influenza panels can develop answers. Left to their own devices, this is unlikely to happen. Groundwork must be done in advance. What is needed is a preliminary breakdown of the decision problem, expressed as a set of derivative questions. Along with the questions there need be agreement on procedures which facilitate the asking and the answering.

On January 30, 1978, for instance, Califano's advisory group did have a set of specific questions. Although the chairman's report is intelligently organized according to the questions, nobody at the meeting forced a systematic and detailed airing of views on each question, one by one. That is the nub, and the rub.

Detailed answers are not treated as the purpose of such meetings. It is not in the tradition of the medical community. Details invoke disagreement. If one foresees a mild pandemic when another thinks that a pandemic, while remote, would be severe, both can agree on immunization without arguing spread or severity. Who wants the argument? Nobody, except perhaps the decision-maker. Even he is likelier than not to feel, when a mild flu impends, that he needs only a consensus on the most general conclusions. But if he wants to lay a base for later review, he will find he also needs the details. He has to insist on their pursuit. Nobody else can or will.

To illustrate the sorts of questions an insistent Mathews or a Cooper might have imposed on advisory committees in March 1976, we have taken a first cut at an appropriate set of questions for the next threat of a severe pandemic. These are included in Appendix E. We think them applicable to any pandemic, although in situations of apparent mildness, like Russian flu, one need not linger long.

The best of expert panels should be supplemented by separate scientific advice. In a swine flu case when evidence is thin—with unobserved phenomena vastly outweighing observations from the three pandemic years of 1918, 1957, 1968 —it is not only the assumptions but appraisal of their scientific quality that top decision-makers need. Panels tend toward "group think" and over-selling, tendencies nurtured by long-standing interchanges and intimacy, as in the influenza fraternity. Other competent scientists, who do not share their group identity or vested interests, should be able to appraise the scientific logic applied to available evidence. In medicine, as in law, there are rules of evidence by which argument can be tested. A Califano needs an assured source of such review to do for him what a good science adviser does for the President. The Secretary may not need one designated "adviser." In medical fields his Department has plenty of scientists. The problem is to make them scrutinize and check each other's logic for his benefit.

In the course of our study we have gained the impression that Califano and his present heads of CDC, NIH (the home of NIAID) and FDA (the home of BoB) have evolved collegial relations close enough and organized enough to test the logic of enthusiasms from below. The Assistant Secretary joins in as a counselor to all. This fivesome seems to work with mutual confidence. If a swine flu case with all its threats and doubts arose today, they probably would talk it out together before writing memoranda to each other. They would do so, at least, if they were not all equally inhibited by bureaucratic stakes or activated by the same professional agendas. Since three of them are linked from underneath, these are substantial qualifications.

This collegium depends on personal relationships. It cannot be a long-term means to give successive Secretaries the reviews they need. It may, however, work for Califano if he takes sufficient pains to induce candor from his colleagues independent of their institutional positions. Otherwise he needs an outside source.

Nowadays if Califano cannot get a check on scientific logic for himself, there is an OSTP to do it, not for him but for Carter. An issue should not rise that high without a test of logic. If it does, however, the President is now somewhat protected. In 1976, had there been an OSTP related to the OMB in current fashion, Ford would not have been dependent on a single, formal meeting of those improvised "advisers" in the Cabinet room. But Califano's needs are not the same as Carter's and cannot be satisfied by OSTP. It does not exist to serve him.

Thus far, advisory panels in the public health field, even including Califano's *ad hoc* groups, have not proceeded in a fashion to assure explicit statements of underlying assumptions, nor has the Secretary yet systematized the science advisory function. We think we understand why. Immunization issues thus far decided in this Administration are so much narrower than Sencer's program of two years ago as almost to defy comparison. The differences stand out: the argument has not run to implementing an unprecedented venture with a palpable effect upon 200 million people. Nor has it run to risking institutions and careers, or other programs. It has not been couched in terms to make senior officials glimpse themselves as heroes; neither has it hinted at a gun to Califano's head. So he has had it easy up to now. What he has seen so far is no assurance that advisory arrangements as they stand will be sufficient in a harder case like swine flu.

Influenza may not be the source of the next hard case. Indeed, it almost surely won't be, unless and until someone foresees another killer wave, another 1918. The flu-ologists have been cooled down. The next hard case is likelier to come from somewhere else and, superficially, seem different.

2. Thinking About Doing

Implementation is not only something to be done after decision, it is as much or more a thing to think about before decision, right along with substance. Of this there was but little in the swine flu case. If Cooper had a tendency to tell himself that he could "doctor his way through," so did almost everyone else.

Had Cooper paused to think about, to ask about, to probe, uncertainties in children's doses, for example, or in production schedules, or in CDC relations with voluntary agencies (to say nothing of medical practitioners), he might have been less cavalier with Young, less content with Meriwether and more cautious about CDC's capacity to manage. Had he paused to contemplate the combination of far more intense surveillance than before with far more people getting shots, he might have promised the health subcommittees less and prepared them better for Legionnaire's Disease, coincident deaths, Guillain-Barré.

The lack of such forethought is no medical monopoly. Had Mathews paused to probe casual assurances that contracts would suffice for liability, he might have warned the President that they had legislation in their laps. This almost surely would have altered much about their consultations, timing and publicity. It also could have raised the spectre of delay in Sencer's schedule, encouraging a close look at his deadlines. It is too much to hope that Mathews might have foreseen the insurance strike (which had never happened before). It would have been enough for him to see that contracting meant foot-dragging by manufacturers, which Kennedy and Rogers had the means to cure—if they chose to cooperate—more surely than Barrett or Feiner.

Even Sencer, urgent as he was once he decided, might have shaped both his decision and his conduct rather differently had he paused to consider dosage problems, ghetto problems, skeptical physicians, media reactions, *and* the fruits of the most serious surveillance ever tried, *if* there were *not* a visible pandemic. The probability of no pandemic was always higher than the chance that there would be one, as Sencer heard from almost everybody except Kilbourne. In combination with these other factors the more likely case held dangers for the credibility of CDC. That should have made Sencer keen to hear what Alexander, from the provinces, was trying to convey. But Sencer seemingly allowed concern over the worst case to obscure thoughts about this likelihood.

In our view a version of Sencer's "minimum response"—with stress upon an idea like "we can't do more until we know more" —would have served the country well even if another swine flu outbreak had occurred. Or his "combined response," the one adopted, could have done it had he made the starting date for his mass immunization contingent on a trigger everyone could understand. If he feared subsequent decisions from a hostile OMB or an electioneering White House, he could have urged preparedness and devised an *automatic* trigger, say a second outbreak of a given size (verified, no doubt, amidst a hullabaloo like the first days of Legionnaire's Disease). Then would have come the time to "doctor through," aided and abetted by the ingenuity of the whole country.

Alternatives like these might have occurred to someone thinking in detail about the do-ability of an all-out response *lacking* another outbreak. With no further sign of swine flu, skeptical states still were unprepared six months after Ford's announcement. Leading skeptics claim to us that they could have both planned and vaccinated (if supplied) within two months had swine flu reappeared. The tort claims bill that Congress put through in a week might still be pending save for

Legionnaire's Disease. Tangibility makes many things more do-able. Its absence is a drag.

Thinking about doing does not happen in a vacuum. It occurs in people's heads and is unlikely to illuminate save as it inter-sects something already there. With 1918 in their heads, let alone 1957, 1968, Sencer and the others presumably would have gone forward anyhow. In March 1976, a positive response of some sort was a sure thing. But more attention to the do-able would almost certainly have altered emphasis and scope. So at least the hopeful light of hindsight makes it seem.

Moreover, what could not be changed could surely have been watched. If not a call to action then a warning for the future would have followed from a look at *operational* assumptions, the assumptions about what, when, how, by whom. To pause over these, and to probe them, can do for implementation what probability analysis and Alexander's question do for substance: lay a base, provide a referent, give a time frame, sound alarms.

Sencer obviously gave *some* thought to do-ability. We argue only that it could have served his purpose (and the public's) to think farther ahead in more detail. His action-memorandum suggests plainly that he thought about the most immediate aspects of implementation: egg supplies, appropriations, plan-ning. The first he sought to meet head on, the second called for circumventing OMB's accustomed stance. His memo shows de-tailed concern for both. The third he meant to improvise with Millar, Seal and Meyer; all were at hand. Perhaps they were too handy. In retrospect, here's where he should have probed de-tails but evidently didn't.

In immediate terms, Sencer gained a tactical advantage by attaching to the manufacturing decision, with its short deadline, the less tightly constrained decision to inoculate. But this de-prived him of strategic opportunities to think through conse-quences of the likely case, the case of no pandemic. And it squeezed down to two weeks the time available for everyone from him through Ford to probe mass immunization before they embraced it.

There are both relatively fancy and quite simple ways to pause and probe the doing before doing it. Engineers learn project management techniques for specifying every forward step. Some schools for public service teach a course on "implementation analysis" which urges students to try mapping *backward* from the last act they intend, identifying prior actions needed as prerequisites. And one of PHS's senior staffers put that exercise to us in simpler guise:

Hell, the thing that was needed in planning the swine flu program was a day around the table brainstorming Murphy's Law: "If anything can go wrong it will"; and all the permutations anyone could think of. That would have done it. It certainly would have caught a lot of the things that went wrong—they weren't so hard to think of, after all.

There are two good times for this. One time is *after* the decision, customarily a period for implementation planning. That time is not at issue. In the swine flu case, Millar and his assistants from their vantage points at CDC did something of the sort (although they certainly were unimaginative about Murphy's Law). The other time, however, is *beforehand*, allowing one to weigh, *in* the decision, estimates of some sort about difficulties, likelihoods and costs of going wrong. But Sencer, though he did this in a way with his own staff, suffered from squinty vision on the public side of management. And Murphy's Law, or backward-mapping, or whatever, was distinctly not pursued by Cooper in advance of his decision. Once *he* decided, it became too late for others to weigh implementation issues very differently.

Cooper's own agenda when the program came along stressed voluntary agencies, practitioners, and parents. We argue that this should have made him sensitive indeed to manifold details of implementation, not least children's dosages, and keen to brainstorm troubles in advance of a decision. But that is an administrator's logic. Cooper was also a doctor. Sencer's validation, once checked out, invoked the absolute regard for life which argued a decision first and details after.

This strikes us as a crucial point. Cooper, the Assistant Secretary for Health, was better placed, by far, than Mathews or the White House to check out Sencer's action-memorandum in these managerial terms, thinking of the doing. But what would have lent weight to Cooper's thoughts was less a matter of administrative status (which could not have stopped insistent agency officials) than of professional standing as perceived in Congress and White House alike. Yet being an M.D., being indeed the only medical practitioner among Assistant Secretaries, he was almost bound to heed the same call Sencer heard: "If we believe in preventive medicine, we have no choice." Why then think farther ahead than Sencer about implementation issues in advance of choice?

Mathews, not a doctor, responded to the same imperative. This left Ford's staff to do the heavy thinking about implementation in advance. Time was short and they were just too far away. Had Mathews seen the issue and his own task differently, his staff might not have been much better off than Ford's.

This leads us to the view that HEW could use an advisory group of political administrators from which panels could be drawn to help Assistant Secretaries and their agency heads think about prospective public interventions. Imagine Cooper or Sencer being asked by Mathews to call in a panel of, say, Manuel Carballo from Wisconsin, Peter Goldmark from New York, Jerald Stevens from Massachusetts, a couple of strong state health commissioners, a couple of local counterparts, one or two sophisticated practicing physicians, all spiced by a manager or two from private life, or even (shades of Rockefeller) from the Pentagon.[36]

This is not at all the sort of body others recommend for an immunization commission. Nor could a commission do what is intended here. The group we now suggest is not meant to be representative of scientists or interests. Neither is it meant to have a scientific mission, nor even a fixed area for oversight. Rather we suggest a reservoir of talent, selected for practical knowledge, not representation, from which panels are drawn when wanted. The panelists should come from places where health interventions actually are carried out. Their purpose is to bring a feel for the intricacies of implementation. Their agendas should be far removed from the routine.

Granting that it would be hard to keep such a group well enough informed for use, and used enough, we think this worth exploring.

3. Thinking of the Media

In the swine flu program, perhaps the greatest defect in the plans for what to do occurred when public health professionals tried thinking about newsmen. There was a glaring lack of institutional connections between medical professionals of every stripe and anybody knowing much of anything about the news profession, above all television news, the primary news source for most Americans. What was at stake amounted less to influencing coverage—in any event hard to do except for fleeting moments—than to anticipating it, preparing for it, weighing in the balance of decision both prospective benefits and costs. In a mass program this is crucial to the thinking about doing. It was badly done.

There was little expertise at hand about the trade of television journalism, to say nothing of production. The Public Information Officer at CDC came out of publishing, not any sort of journalism, although he was conscientious in his services to journalists, which is what he should be. Sencer and Cooper were part of a medical generation unused to having its motives questioned. Meyer and Seal looked back to 1957, the first year "television homes" began to rival "radio homes," a far-gone age in television's history. Cavanaugh and O'Neill, politicized bureaucrats both, had less than infallible instincts, and anyway did not have the *time* to sharpen them up; network news was televised during their working hours. Some of Mathews' aides may have had glimmerings; Cooper walled them off. The Information Officer in PHS is said to have been street-wise; he was not consulted.

Still, however thin the in-house expertise on media reactions, experts in influenza made almost no effort to secure it or improve on it. They evidently saw no need. They may not have conceived that there was anything they lacked. In all events, they acted as though journalists were (or should be) but conveyor belts for medical professionals, with no professionalism of their own or none, at any rate, worth deference from doctors. There followed one egregious error after another. When Sencer shoved a technical consensus somewhat past its freely given limits, inside CDC and out, he was asking for leaks from insiders and defections from advisers. How could they resist TV? It was almost sure to come their way. Controversy spices life on television news, prized by producers, hence by reporters, built into their incentives, bound to be pursued on the occasion of White House announcements in election years. By the same token, Cavanaugh should have strained to assure himself of Sencer's troops, especially the younger generation closest to the lab, those likeliest to be in love with their experiments more than with Sencer's policies.

In June, to take another instance, Sencer argued that Americans identify immunization with their children and that an announcement giving up on children was unthinkable so early in the day. Well and good, but better had the thought occurred in March when there was time to do something about it.

Later in the day, for a third instance, someone at CDC should have remembered early talk of temporally related deaths, and been prepared for Pittsburgh. A Pittsburgh almost had to come and surely should have been rehearsed in early consultation with the states. While negligent production, a "bad batch," was an alternative cause until ruled out, this only is to say that states should have been briefed on both alternatives. What was most damaging in news announcements were the hesitant and variable reactions in the states. These might have been blunted or avoided. They might, that is to say, had the anticipation of such coverage been anybody's business, or more precisely that of anybody with some talent for it.

Still later, the public problem posed by Guillain-Barré syndrome—inability to state the risk for a consent form—need not have taken unawares anyone who bothered to consider Hattwick's search for side effects, the unknowns he expected to trace. Some members of the public health community consider it a moral outrage that, with Hattwick's expectations, the program was allowed to proceed. Since the side effect discovered can be estimated now at one fatality in some two million, we ourselves eschew the moral issue. But the operational issue, what to do with something new while risks are under study, could have been faced earlier. The issue never surfaced in advance at CDC; not arising there, it could not arise at higher levels.

A Califano should be able to build links between medical specialists and advisers who can help them come to better terms with television news. Their need is to stop thinking about "shoulds" (TV *should* convey our message as *we* conceive it) and to start thinking about what can reasonably be expected from the medium in given cases, assuming both reporters and producers do decent work in *their* profession's terms. On that standard we find relatively little to complain of and some things to admire in our sampling of the swine flu TV coverage.[37] As the Secretary deals with public health officials, he has either to make doctors appreciate electronic journalism, a hard job, or to help the Assistant Secretary and his agency chiefs instill some good sense about television into their advisory system. Daily news reporters and producers cannot serve. Corporate executives don't substitute. Trade associations are not in point. Thoughtful politicians or reporters once-removed from daily news are needed. Seeding one or two into the panels of political administrators we propose might have a large effect. Could a Moyers be borrowed? Is a Sevareid wholly retired?

Unlike most Federal departments, HEW because of size decentralizes press operations. The Assistant Secretary for Public Affairs and the press officer of the Department serve the Secretary. They review all releases nowadays (a change from 1976), but PHS and CDC still have their own press offices. In a swine flu case, unprecedented, urgent, national in scope, the departmental staff seems better placed than others to anticipate reactions by and through the media. It is better placed because it deals more regularly than others with reporters on the beat from networks, wire services and national newspapers. Although more sparsely covered than the Pentagon or White House, HEW is now a beat; the daily work of journalists on national news stories should be known there. But departmental staff—also that of PHS—was on the sidelines in the swine flu case. Judging from the early struggle over organization, this had not been Mathews' intention. It was, however, the effect of Cooper's preemption. The *ad hoc* press officer for swine flu became Meriwether, who had everything to learn.

4. Maintaining Credibility

One of the things at stake in media relations was the credibility of Ford's expert advisers with attentive publics: medical, political and press circles alike, and influential citizens from other walks of life who helped to set the tone of wider groups. The President could offer visibility, but in his circumstances as a primary campaigner he had no credibility to spare; indeed his needs ran the other way—he had to borrow. Those he borrowed from were on the one hand individuals established in their own careers, like Salk or for that matter Cooper, and on the other hand the agencies established in the field of public health, like CDC.

The swine flu program put the latter's reputation on the line. This, remarkably, was not at Ford's initiative. Rather it was the doing of the agency's director. Still more remarkably, neither Sencer nor his bosses, Cooper, Mathews, Ford, seem to have considered whether there was need for this or what might be its cost.

Two years later, mortgaging the reputation of the CDC to swine flu does seem costly. As the science reporter for a TV network commented to us:

CDC was almost the last Federal agency widely regarded by reporters and producers as a *good thing*, responsible, respectable, scientific, above suspicion. This gave Sencer terrific clout. The Presidency after Watergate, the military after Vietnam, physicists, universities, to say nothing of HEW or Congress for God's sake—none of them remotely in the same league! Even a hint that any one of them was blocking Sencer's urgent memo would have been a big story . . . human interest . . . good guys (the best) against bad. . . . Now CDC's lost its innocence. . . .

The innocence has gone, and with it clout, not for all time, as memories fade and new impressions take hold (if they do), but for some years. The loser is not likely to be CDC as such but rather new departures in preventive medicine. When it espouses these it almost surely will be tagged as crying "wolf."

If CDC should happen to foresee correctly the next public

health disaster, then its loss of status may affect the lives of citizens. That was and is the reason for concern about its reputation in the longer run. What is to us remarkable is that, so far as we can find, no one from Sencer up gave this a thought (and those below who did, or now believe they did, were brushed aside).

Here, we think, was a missed opportunity, indeed two opportunities in one. Sencer concentrated on the worst case in the shortest run. So did his superiors. Had they thought equally hard about the likely case in the longer run—side effects and suits but no pandemic—the issue of diminished credibility for CDC would have loomed large, hard to ignore. Or had they started at the other end by thinking about CDC's prospective reputation, this should have made the likely case stand out against the worst: the likely case might very well be harder on the agency. Either mode of thought leads toward the other. Both induce concern about the role of CDC. Both pile up doubts about the role that Sencer chose, the super-salesman's role.

Had Sencer posed the issues candidly, with the uncertainties spelled out, the likelihoods compared, deadlines unscrambled and production his immediate concern, the credibility of CDC would now be better than it is. Had he not sought control of operations it would be still better.

Cooper and the laymen in their turn performed just as had Sencer, buying his argument, selling the next echelon. This did not help CDC preserve its innocence, but does add to our sympathy for Sencer. Everybody *wanted* to be sold.

To tie the reputation of an agency to short-term fears (or hopes) was not Sencer's invention. On the contrary, it is an everyday affair, at least in Washington. Sencer has plenty of company, some of it presidential. Nixon risked the reputation of the White House itself. Others have been cavalier with institutions more removed—Johnson's escalation of the Vietnam war was classic in its consequences for the Army, one of many. Presidents, of course, are at the center of the storm, struggling with irreconcilable expectations while claiming the legitimacy of national election. They and their fellow politicians on the Hill are supposedly responsible for balancing short-run and long.

Their judgment, within limits, has the sanction of our constitutional system.

Sencer was not President. Yet as he did his work this may be a distinction without a difference. For he evidently thought it was his task to make his constitutional superiors do right no matter what they thought (and so he did). He also made them do it with but little time to think.

Legitimation by election, the embodiment of popular sovereignty, is a far cry from legitimation by professional training and consultation. The first is a political value, the second a scientific one. Not even *pro forma* is there any means to reconcile the two. Unlike the military, medical professionals do not have in their value system a ready rationale like "commander-in-chief." Sencer pushed his bosses without stint. They were his constitutional superiors but that gave him no pause. Cooper aside, they were laymen. Sencer evidently held the not uncommon premise that the boobs could not be trusted to decide right on their own.

This we believe is what made him a salesman. On that premise he could not afford to take the opportunity we say he missed, could not allow himself to dawdle over either of the questions we propose—neither what's the likely case over a longer time, nor what's the risk to CDC's reputation. Had he pursued them, either one, he soon would have been led to the more open stance of a technician serving up to his superiors the data for *their* judgment. We think this stance both prudent for his agency and proper in his role. Plainly he did not think so.

As a prerequisite to playing the technician's role, a man in Sencer's shoes has to accept the notion that the politicians may be boobs but it is they who were elected.

5. Thinking Twice About Medical Knowledge

We have called influenza a "slippery" disease. Five features combine to make it so.

First is the changing character of the influenza virus, with spread and timing mortgaged to the processes of antigenic change about which there are painfully few documented observations. As for severity, the specialists are almost wholly in the dark. Nothing is sure, not even the reasons why 1918 was the worst flu of all.

Second, the effectiveness of influenza vaccine is relatively short-lived. Its effectiveness may be compromised by minor antigenic drifts in the virus, which are frequent. Moreover, most experts believe that, even in the absence of drift, effective protection lasts only for about a year.

Third, influenza symptoms are widely misunderstood. Millions of Americans, and perhaps half the doctors in the country, use the term for a variety of gastrointestinal troubles, "stomach flu," which no flu virus causes and no flu vaccine cures. Influenza virus is found predominantly in the respiratory tract.

Fourth, although it resides in the respiratory tract, it is by no means the only virus likely to be lurking there and may not be the major source of flu-like aches and fever. If not, then immunization against influenza, even assuming that the vaccine fits the strain and that it actually immunizes, safeguards nobody from identical symptoms caused by other viruses.

Fifth, the multitude of causes of flu-like illness make it difficut to estimate the year-to-year impact of the influenza virus on the public health. Especially in non-epidemic years, the proportion of flu-like illness actually caused by the flu virus is unknown.

We elaborate on these five features in our Technical Afterword.

Without more evidence of swine flu's spread than Sencer had in March 1976, consider how these features mock his objectives, and Cooper's. What a basis on which to build public consciousness and to seek support for preventive medicine! What a basis on which to risk the high repute of an establishment like CDC! What a basis, for that matter, on which to expose 40 million people to an unknown risk of side effects! And all this on the word of experts, overconfident in theories validated through but two or three pandemics, without any proper review of their logic by disinterested scientists. It is not that conclusions were inconsistent with evidence, but that the paucity of evidence belied the force with which conclusions were advanced.

Contrast influenza's features with those of well-established

Federal immunization targets, measles and polio, or smallpox in its day. For the established targets, causes, symptoms, treatments, risks are understood alike by doctors and laymen. Immunization "immunizes": it prevents the symptoms for all time, or for several years at least. From decade to decade there are no antigenic shifts. Compared to the slippery flu, these are stable targets indeed. Medical and public health professionals, congressmen, administrators, parents, children, journalists and citizens at large all know what they are shooting at.

The comparative aspect is critical. All diseases are slippery in some degree. All interventions risk, to some degree, the credibility of institutions. But to treat swine flu as though it were the polio of twenty years ago is to beg for trouble. The two diseases have some tempting likenesses but in these key respects they are at opposite ends of the spectrum. When this country started on its campaign against polio it confronted a well-understood disease with methods that worked as advertised. Contrast the swine flu program. It oversold a method of ostensible protection from the paradigm of slippery diseases. The risk to credibility was rendered as extreme as was the combination of its five slippery features.

Up to 1976, the Federal government had drawn a line, perhaps unconsciously, between stable and such slippery diseases. Swine flu represented the first Federally sponsored and financed mass immunization at the slippery end of the spectrum. Diseases at the stable end had been an exclusive company. Its members shared an inferential base of medical knowledge, public understanding, and support, far beyond that now accorded influenza. On the evidence of swine flu, it is tempting to propose a restoration of the former line, and consciously bar slippery diseases, flu included, from Federal immunization initiatives. The stress would be on research until they were rendered less slippery.

This may fit other slippery diseases, but not flu. In contrast with the common cold and possibly some cancers, influenza has one very solid facet: specific preventives that precisely match some demonstrable risks of death. Where risks are high and counter-measures readily available, exceptions must be made to any bar against the slippery diseases.

Still, we would hedge such exceptions tightly. The risk should be of death. The preventive available should be effective for those people most at risk. It should substantially increase their chances of survival. For flu vaccine this means the right strength, matching the right virus with the right number of doses, deliverable in good time, and properly administered to those whose risk of death is so severe as to outweigh the disadvantages of public intervention. With flu as slippery as it now is, those disadvantages are weighty. Countervailing risk of death should not be assigned loosely to large populations.

Workers who are not at risk of death may be greatly convenienced by the same vaccine. At this stage of medical knowledge, they and their physicians and employers are the ones we think should judge whether benefits of vaccination outweigh disadvantages. They, not public health officials, should decide and their budgets, not those of public health, should bear the cost (except perhaps for local services like fire or police).

Under national health insurance this judgment might change. But it would then be a judgment for the health authorities to make in allocating limited dollars among competing treatments for different diseases. As in the Canadian case two years ago, influenza treatments might be limited. But national insurance is another story.

The proposed Federal program directed against Russian flu strikes us as not far out of line with our exception and its stated limits. Including everybody over 65, however healthy, has an odd ring in the first year of a raised retirement age, now 70. Age alone, apart from other illnesses, may prove a lesser factor in flu deaths than has been thought. Aside from this the program seems appropriately modest. But its very modesty may be in part an accident of circumstances. So long as liability issues are unresolved, Federal policy can scarcely go beyond financing state procurement of vaccine for limited numbers of people, few enough to keep down fears of lawsuits in the skittish minds of manufacturers and insurers. The risk of death is such a natural, traditional criterion, appealing to and understood by all, that we are confident it will prevail whenever numbers must be limited. But if and when a comprehensive liability solution comes to pass, then all too easily the definitions of "high-risk" could be progressively relaxed, and we would lose our tight tie between preventive and risk of death.

Judging from the swine flu story this is precisely what one should expect to follow upon liability legislation.

Thus we do not think that our criterion of matching risk to preventive will suffice for long to limit influenza's claims upon the once exclusive club of Federal immunization initiatives. How then maintain the limit while researchers try to improve understanding of flu's other facets?

The obvious answer is budgeting. Federal expenditures for purchase and delivery of flu vaccine should stand on their own merits, in competition with other Federal programs. But which other programs? We are not now in a position to advise on the appropriate arena for that competition. It clearly would be wrong if CDC alone were made to fund progressive intervention in the influenza sphere out of the other programs in its budget. At the other extreme it may be wrong for influenza to compete with everything else in Federal health.[38] Yet some competitive arena ought to be delineated. What is assuredly wrong is to have no competition at all.

That is the current condition, fortuitously veiled by liability.

In general, restricting the exceptions for a slippery disease to risk of death limits the scope of Federal intervention. However, in one circumstance, this same criterion would open the door wide to virtually unlimited immunization against influenza. That is the coming of another "killer" wave, another 1918. This is what was feared in 1976. But the threat was never established. We believe that in the absence of *manifest* danger, all-out action was a mistake. One can, of course, start manufacturing more vaccine at the first hint of a killer. But one cannot reasonably stick it into people without more concrete evidence than anybody had at any time in 1976. To do so is to court medical dissent, to spread public confusion, and to provoke suspicion in the Washington community. Since research has not yet found a good predictor of virulence, one may have no means to establish in advance the severity of a presumed pandemic. Establishing that 1918 has come back again means waiting for manifestations somewhere in the world, maybe here. There is no way around it. Somewhere in the world, some people have to die.

That is a challenge to medical research: how to predict virulence before the virus strikes.

For influenza, virulence and many other technical questions are important not only for future research, but also because current policy decisions turn on answers, or at least on expert guesses at the answers. Our next task, and the last in this study, is to sketch some of the technical dilemmas posed by flu; first, those related to the virus and disease, and second, those related to prevention and control. This we do in our Afterword. To the degree research unravels these dilemmas, influenza will become a far less slippery disease.

13

TECHNICAL

AFTERWORD

Policy decisions regarding influenza rest on judgments about the behavior of the virus, the impact of the disease and our ability to interdict its course. But the virus is capricious, the disease elusive, and our remedies imperfect. The technical dilemmas discussed in this Afterword reflect what we know, what we think we know and what we do not know. They run from matters of definition, to matters of measurement, to matters of substantive understanding. We hope they convey the nature of technical limitations in contending with the influenza problems.

Influenza Virus and Disease

The term influenza applies both to a particular virus and to a clinical disease, consisting of fever, headache, muscle aches, prostration and, frequently, cough, watery eyes, nasal stuffiness. The influenza virus can cause this syndrome, although not always exactly the same symptoms, and the severity of the disease ranges from very mild to fatal; death usually comes from rapidly progressive pneumonia.[39]

Many other infectious agents, mostly viruses, can produce illness resembling that caused by the influenza virus.[40] Influenza-the-virus certainly predominates as a cause of influenza-the-disease during epidemic periods, but other viruses are relatively more prominent as producers of year-in and year-out influenza-like illness. Persons who are vaccinated and protected against the influenza virus remain susceptible to "flu" when caused by other organisms.

Public understanding thus is constantly at risk. To virologists and influenza experts, "influenza" means the influenza virus and only the disease produced by that virus. To members of the public, "flu" is the disease regardless of viral cause. Many people also speak colloquially of "intestinal flu," a misnomer to the specialist since influenza is not a gastrointestinal ailment.

For public policy, therefore, the problem of influenza-the-disease is analytically distinct from problems produced by the influenza virus. This applies to any assessment of the health and economic magnitude of the "influenza" problem, to the development of short- and long-term strategies to address the "influenza" problem, and to the presentation and promotion of "influenza" programs.

The significance of influenza-the-virus to national health is substantial, but the measures used to assess its importance have many limitations. The medical consequences of illness can be described in terms of mortality, or deaths, and morbidity, or discomfort and disability. In estimating the morbidity and mortality due to influenza virus, two main difficulties arise. First, because of the overlap in clinical symptoms produced by different infectious agents, estimates of influenza-like illness would overstate the effects of the influenza virus. (The degree of exaggeration depends on the relative prevalence of other viruses at the time the estimate is made.) Second, influenza viruses not only cause death directly and in association with bacterial pneumonia, but very often may contribute to death in patients with other, serious primary illnesses, such as heart, lung and renal disease. In fact, during a typical year, the "influenza-related" deaths due primarily to other diseases are believed to outnumber those directly due to influenza and pneumonia.[41]

In order to detect the occurrence of influenza epidemics and to capture their full impact on mortality, the CDC has for years relied on a derived index, called "excess mortality." Mortality rates normally show a regular year-round fluctuation, highest in winter and lowest in summer. The CDC currently receives weekly mortality counts (total deaths and those attributed to pneumonia and influenza) from 121 urban centers around the country, comprising about 30 percent of the U.S. population. The CDC compares the observed mortality with the "normal" curve, which is based on a composite of several years' experience. If the reported mortality exceeds a certain threshold for two consecutive weeks, this is considered indicative of an epidemic. CDC sums the number of excess deaths reported by the 121 cities during the flu season (usually 2–3 months), computes an "excess mortality" rate per 100,000 population covered, and then extrapolates to the entire population to derive a total number of excess deaths in the country.[42]

Computation of excess mortality is a sensitive way to identify the occurrence of an epidemic, but it may be an inaccurate indicator of influenza's importance as a national health problem. First, urban centers, having relatively dense concentrations of people, would be more likely to experience epidemic outbreaks; extrapolating from 70 million city dwellers to the entire country may therefore exaggerate national experience. Second, restricting the excess death counts to the influenza season fails to correct for those patients who would have died shortly (within the year) without any influenza. One old study concluded this effect was present, but small, and that most excess deaths occurred in people who were not just about to die anyway.[43] A recent comparison of CDC's calculated excess mortality with annual mortality data compiled by the National Center for Health Statistics (NCHS) suggests that CDC's excess mortality estimates have tended to be too high in recent years.[44]

In addition to possible inaccuracies of this sort, the number of deaths is an incomplete measure of the importance of influenza virus as a cause of death. For purposes of setting priorities among health programs, a vital, supplementary measure is the "years of life lost" due to disease.[45] This is a function of both mortality rate and age at death. Everyone is going to die, and what is important is not the fact of death, but its prematurity, the number of years of life expectancy foreclosed. This could be calculated from age-specific death rates compiled on an annual basis. But so far as we know, the calculation has not been done by CDC. Therefore, its attributions of mortality cannot be adjusted in this way. Elderly persons make up such a high proportion of influenza deaths that the adjustment could reduce flu's relative importance as a cause of death in this country.

A further limitation to the CDC's "excess mortality" measure is its inability to reflect the extent of *non*-fatal influenza. No mortality measure, even if otherwise perfect, can do that. The extent of temporarily disabling influenza can be decidedly important to employers and school superintendents alike, also of course to the patient. This, too, is an aspect of influenza's standing among national health problems. Indeed, the NCHS does count in its weekly household surveys the number of influenza-like illnesses in the population.[46] But that is just the difficulty. These measures cannot distinguish flu from other things that have the same effects on people. Catch-22!

The extent and severity of illness caused by the influenza virus appears to depend on characteristics of the virus, of people at risk of infection, and of the environment. Scientific understanding of the contribution of each is incomplete.

The influenza virus contains eight genetic fragments. This arrangement of genetic material into separate segments is unusual among viruses. When the influenza virus invades a host cell its genes commandeer the cell's machinery and synthesize seven proteins incorporated into the virus and a couple which are left in the host cell.[47] Two of those virus proteins are internal antigens, by which the virus can be typed as A, B or C (in descending order of importance to humans). Two are the surface antigens, H (Hemagglutinin) and N (Neuraminidase), which undergo the major "shifts" and minor "drifts" that camouflage the virus to a host's antibodies. Shifts are attributed to the reassortment of gene segments from two different influenza viruses. This primitive form of sexual reproduction results in a recombinant virus which has some properties of each parent. Drifts are believed due to mutation in a single gene.[48]

As a matter of convention, influenza viruses are named according to a system adopted by the World Health Organization in 1971. The strain designation includes the antigenic type (A, B or C), the species from which the strain was first isolated (if non-human), the country or city where it was first found, its laboratory strain number and the year of isolation. In addition, for type A viruses, its specific H and N antigens may be cited, usually in parentheses following the strain designation. The swine flu virus, for example, was formally named A/New Jersey/8/76 (Hsw1N1).[49]

Each antigenic shift to a new H or N antigen, or both, produces a new subtype of the virus. Type A subtypes now active include H1N1 (A/Russian) and H3N2 (A/Victoria). Within each subtype, there may be further variations caused by antigenic drifts. A/Texas, for example, drifted from A/Victoria; both are H3N2 viruses. For simplicity, we have used only place names in our narrative. There we deal only with type A flu, since that type alone is believed to cause pandemics.[50]

Regarding the flu viruses, little is known about the determinant of infectivity (ability to invade cells and cause illness), mobility (ability to spread from person to person) or virulence (ability to cause serious disease and death). To further complicate matters, the greater the number of virus particles to which a person is exposed at one time, other things equal, the more likely is illness to follow. Attempts to test a new virus strain in human volunteers can give misleading results because laboratory passage of the virus may have attenuated its virulence.[51]

Different individuals are differently susceptible to infection and to complications from infection. Individual resistance to infection is related to a person's level of antibodies to the infecting virus. School-age children, especially age 5–14 years, are most commonly affected by influenza. Patients debilitated by other medical conditions are more likely to die from influenza than are healthy persons. Infants and the elderly are likelier to die than young adults (although the great pandemic of 1918 also killed many of them). These likelihoods rest on statistical associations and call for close scrutiny. Since so many flu-related deaths involve other diseases, either the virus has profound effects on healthy tissue outside the lungs or other illnesses contribute in a major way to deaths "from" influenza. Thus the statistical association of those deaths with age may actually reflect not years as such, but rather other illnesses common among the elderly. A healthy oldster may be little or no more likely to die from flu than a healthy young adult.

Death from influenza is rare overall (less than 0.1 percent of cases), but mortality from a nationwide epidemic can be in the tens of thousands because of the enormous numbers afflicted. The large number of deaths attributed to the Asian flu in 1957 (more than 60,000) is probably due to the very high attack rate, and not to any unusual virulence of the virus.[52]

Environmental effects, including biological, physical and social factors, can also alter the course of influenza. For reasons which are not understood, epidemic influenza is a seasonal illness in temperate climates.[53] Concomitant bacterial infection in individual patients can produce serious complications. A closed setting, such as a boarding school, nursing home or military base is conducive to the spread of disease. Indeed, experience at Fort Dix in 1976 emphasizes the hazards of projecting to the general community observation of viral spread in a closed community, where crowding and stress prevail.

One additional phenomenon is worth noting here: the second wave of a particular virus subtype occasionally causes more deaths than the first wave. This was true of the 1918 pandemic worldwide, of the 1968–70 Hong Kong epidemics in Europe, and possibly of the 1889–90 Asiatic influenza.[54] It is not clear whether a particular virus may attain increased infectivity or virulence over time, whether some people become sensitized and overreact to subsequent infection or whether there is some other explanation.

Predictions of the severity and extent of influenza-the-virus in any given year are very shaky. In particular, speculations about periodicity of influenza pandemics rest on a slender factual base. Epidemiologists are largely confined to natural experiments, to the observed occurrence of influenza epidemics in the human population. Only since the 1930's have we had techniques for isolating and identifying viruses. Recognition of influenza subtypes came later. Since then there have been only a few influenza pandemics, a few observations with a relatively long time to discuss them and to theorize about them. Serological evidence can extend knowledge of previous epidemics back to the births of living individuals, but this offers at best a few more observations.

Long reflection on a limited number of observations has given rise to such conventional dogmas as the cyclical appearance of pandemics every decade or so.

Influenza pandemics are worldwide occurrences of disease, while epidemics are lesser but still wide-spread outbreaks. One careful historical review identified ten definite pandemics and ten possible pandemics in the past 250 years (not including this year's Russian flu).[55] The intervals between definite pandemics varied from 10 to 49 years, 24 years on average, and the intervals between all twenty definite or possible pandemics varied from 3 to 28 years, a 12-year average. Thus, pandemics have occurred at very irregular intervals, and the average interpandemic period has been between 12 and 24 years.

In addition to the questionable theory of regular pandemic cycles, there is a separate theory that influenza A has a limited number of subtypes which recycle through the human population.[56] This theory holds that subtypes reappear every other generation as those immunized by previous exposure die off, leaving a huge pool of susceptible people. The regularity of reappearance is questionable.[57] Old viruses can turn up again —witness this year's Russian virus, the same subtype as the virus prevalent (with minor drifts) from 1947 to 1957. Sadly for the theory, and maybe for the virus, it returned in just one generation.

Circumstantial evidence supports the idea that antigenic shifts in human influenza are due to recombinants of animal and human viruses.[58] The theory is that a human core gains animal surface antigens. Such a recombinant event, producing an antigenic shift, is believed prerequisite to worldwide pandemic. This is among the reasons why swine flu was taken so seriously when it reappeared in humans after many years in pigs.

Epidemic extent and severity (as measured by excess mortality) do not correspond in any simple way with antigenic changes in the virus. Experience with the Fort Dix virus reconfirms a few earlier observations that new antigenic strains isolated in humans do not necessarily take hold in the population.[59] We do not yet know enough to predict which new strains will take hold and which won't. Since viruses were first isolated in the 1930's, the only universally acknowledged antigenic shifts with wide effects on people came in 1957 (39 years after 1918), 1968 (11 years after 1957) and in 1977–78 (9 years after 1968). The 1947 virus is considered a shift by some and the product of a sequence of drifts by others.[60] Since the mid-1930's, the greatest "excess mortality" in the United States attributed to influenza occurred in the years 1937, 1943, 1953, 1957 and 1960, only one of which (1957) was also the year a shift occurred and pandemic ensued. In 1968, also a year of antigenic shift, there was less mortality than occurred in the other years listed.[61]

The lack of correspondence between antigenic shifts and excess mortality punctures a traditional piece of conventional wisdom. The new conventional wisdom, becoming current since the swine flu affair, is that flu mortality is not alone or even mainly a problem of pandemics.[62] It is now seen to center in the frequent epidemics, which occur every one to three years.

Prevention and Control

There is no completely effective and safe way to guard a population against influenza virus. The principal means which have been proposed are vaccines and drugs.

Traditional teaching in medicine's antibiotic era has been that bacterial disease is treatable, but there are no good drugs against viruses. This is no longer true, at least not for all viruses. The drug amantadine appears to be effective in preventing type A influenza, and some believe it will also shorten the course of illness.[63] A few physicians advocate its use during flu season, especially for high-risk patients.[64] However, it is dismissed as an "impractical" intervention by others in part because of questions regarding its efficacy and in part because of side effects.[65] These side effects are mainly mild central nervous system reactions such as dizziness, insomnia and confusion, and while uncommon at recommended dosages, occur more often in the elderly. Some physicians have extensive experience with amantadine, but it has not been used on a scale large enough and time period short enough to detect unanticipated, very rare side effects. To be an effective preventive, amantadine must be used daily and would cost approximately 50 cents per day or roughly the same as a single dose of vaccine good for an entire season. Despite its uncertainties and drawbacks, amantadine deserves serious consideration, at least as an adjunct measure, in planning for influenza epidemics.[66]

Research is also under way on other antiviral agents, such as interferon, a naturally produced substance which inhibits viral invasion of cells. As additional information accumulates, and possibly as new drugs are identified, reliable antiviral agents are likely to become more important weapons to counter influenza in the future. If and as they do, the roles of the FDA and private sector probably will increase relative to those of CDC and the state health departments. Tensions may impend in and among agencies, to say nothing of researchers with different agendas.

Naturally acquired influenza stimulates many of the body's defenses against subsequent infection: local defense cells gear up, secretory antibodies coat the respiratory tract and serum antibodies circulate in the blood. Vaccination, by contrast, primarily produces a rise in specific, circulating antibody. This is sufficient to provide some protection, but the quality of immunity differs from that following natural infection.[67] Both anti-hemagglutinin and anti-neuraminidase antibodies contribute to resistance from infection. However, the former is much more protective than the latter.[68]

Vaccination strategies differ for different diseases. In smallpox eradication, for example, the idea was to contain disease by vaccinating people in the immediate vicinity of any new cases. In another instance, children are vaccinated against rubella (German measles) so they will not carry disease to their pregnant mothers. Some vaccination programs aim at herd immunity, achieved by vaccinating enough people to suppress epidemic spread in a population. Some have advocated this approach for influenza.[69] However, herd immunity does not seem reliable for influenza at achievable levels of immunization in the population.[70] Outbreaks have spread in boarding schools, even when more than 95 percent had been vaccinated.[71] Therefore, advocates of influenza vaccination usually stress protection for the individual against the virus and its consequences, without regard for herd effect. This was the prevailing view at CDC in 1976 and is so now. Civilian immunization programs typically focus on the groups at increased risk of death; for example, the elderly and the chronically ill. Military forces try to prevent illness in large numbers of their troops at the same time.

Both live and killed virus vaccines are used in different countries to prevent influenza. Live vaccine has certain theoretical advantages, including protection more akin to that from natural infection and lower volume of virus required for immunization, but questions about its dependability, safety and acceptability (it must be inhaled) have thus far discouraged its use in the United States.[72] Over the near term, killed virus vaccine will probably remain the key element in programs to control influenza in the United States.

Insofar as scientists can more quickly produce more potent vaccines against a broader spectrum of strains, longer-lasting and with fewer side effects, we will strengthen our hand against the influenza virus. No strategy against the virus, no matter how successful, copes with the whole "influenza" disease problem.

In the remainder of this section, we will touch upon vaccine production and side effects, both highlighted in the swine flu story, and then discuss technical issues related to vaccine effectiveness.

Producing vaccine entails a series of connected steps.[73] The first two are isolation of the virus and preparation of recombinant strains. Kilbourne pioneered recombinant technique.[74] His laboratory still sets standards and has customarily prepared recombinant strains for vaccine production, as with swine flu. The next steps are seed lot preparation, growth of vaccine (in enough embryonated eggs), inactivation, purification and concentration in bulk. This is where the manufacturers paused in the summer of 1976. The last steps are dilution to required strength and packaging.

What matters in production is not only the time until the first dose of vaccine is ready for testing, but also the rate and volume at which vaccine is produced thereafter. Technical improvements in any stage may speed production of the first dose, but the volume of output can be rapidly expanded only by widening a choke-point. That point, we are told by laboratory specialists for one manufacturer, is the purification process. Research to prepare for intensive production in the future should focus on such points. They, not facilities in general, limit production.

Rare side effects can be detected only by a comprehensive and sensitive surveillance system. These are unlikely to reveal themselves during field trials. Whether side effects such as Guillain-Barré syndrome are related only to swine flu vaccines, or to any influenza vaccine, or to any vaccine of any kind, is not now known.

The effectiveness of flu vaccines in the general population remains uncertain. Despite administration of millions of doses of vaccine, there have been no direct measures of the extent to which immunization reduces mortality. In terms of ability to prevent disease, the measured effectiveness of influenza vaccines has ranged in different studies from zero to 100 percent.[75] The expert consensus is that present influenza vaccines would be about 60 to 80 percent effective in the general population.[76] By this is meant that compared to an unvaccinated group, 60 to 80 percent fewer people in a similar but vaccinated group will contract influenza.

There are many determinants of vaccine effectiveness and of differences in measured effectiveness.

One of these is variability in the amount and potency of antigen in supposedly equivalent vaccines. Up until this year, the standard vaccine content was measured in CCA (chick cell agglutination) units. However, CCA directly measures only the biologic activity of one viral protein and not its immunologic activity, nor does it reflect the amount of antigen in a dose of vaccine. This shortcoming is well recognized, and work has been done at NIAID and BoB to develop a better standard of measurement for antigenic amounts. The question of antigenic potency (ability to stimulate antibody response) for a given amount of antigen is particularly important because of the different types of killed vaccine produced by different manufacturers—some using whole viruses and some using chemically split viruses. Whole virus preparation and split virus vaccines both have their advocates, the first because of potency and the second because of lessened reactivity. Other, more subtle differences in manufacturing technique may also affect vaccine potency.

Healthy persons will differ in their antibody response to equally potent doses of vaccine, depending on age and previous exposure to this or similar antigens. There will also be normal biologic variation in antibody response among persons of similar age and antigenic history. In persons who have never been previously exposed to a particular viral antigen, often the case with children, it may take two separate injections, the first used as a "priming" dose, to stimulate adequate antibody response.[77]

In general, resistance to influenza virus increases as specific antibody level rises, but level of antibody is not the sole factor in protection from the virus.[78] Changes in the infectivity of the virus, differences in numbers of invading organisms, alterations in the biological, physical or social environment can all affect the likelihood of illness in an individual who has a given level of circulating antibody.

Antibody is most reactive with the specific antigen which prompted its production. However, there is often some degree of cross-reactivity with similar antigens. To the extent that influenza viruses in the field undergo antigenic drift, or that the seed virus preparation and vaccine production alter the antigenic content of the vaccine, immunization effectiveness will be compromised.

Variation in the interval between vaccination and exposure to the virus will also affect the degree of protection. Two or more weeks must pass before a person produces adequate antibody to an injected antigen. The duration of protection from a shot of influenza vaccine is controversial, but there probably is some decline in protection after about six months.[79] Part of the reason for disagreement is that those who believe in longer-term protection attribute rising attack rates to antigenic drift in the virus.

Different methods for assessing vaccine effectiveness can produce differences in apparent efficacy. These include methods of testing and surveillance as well as the criteria for diagnosis.[80] All ways to assess vaccine depend on differences in disease rates between vaccinated and unvaccinated. Thus the incidence of influenza must reach a rather substantial level before differences can be detected. Testing and surveillance wait on that. Problems with diagnosis are related to the fact that flu-like illnesses may not be caused by influenza viruses. If the clinical syndrome alone is considered indicative of influenza, the apparent efficacy of vaccine will decline; infection by other agents, unaffected by the vaccine, will be counted against it. Laboratory identification of the influenza virus would solve that, but isolation of the virus is too inconsistent among cases to be useful in assessing vaccine effectiveness. Clinicians often rely on a four-fold rise in antibody level, from before to after illness, to show infection by a particular agent. But the usual antibody rise in response to infection may be stifled by recent vaccination. Hence, persons genuinely ill from flu soon after getting shots might not be counted as cases of influenza; apparent vaccine efficacy then would rise higher than it was in fact.

Finally, observed vaccine effectiveness in one population may not apply to others. Findings in the military may not apply to civilian populations; findings in nursing homes may not apply to the elderly living on their own; and findings in one age group may not apply to another.

Taken together, the foregoing comments elaborate, selectively, the five features of influenza we set forth in Chapter 12: first, a capricious virus; second, short-lived (and partial) protection against it; third, attribution to it of assorted other ailments; fourth, a mimicking by others of its symptoms; and as a consequence, the fifth, entanglement of influenza-the-virus with influenza-the-disease, causing confusion in the measurement of impact. These are the features that, taken together, give influenza standing in our eyes as an extremely slippery phenomenon.

Regarding swine flu, one question remains to be asked. In 1918, something extraordinary happened: Why? What accounts for the most devastating influenza pandemic history records? Why were young, healthy adults carried off as surely as the elderly and infirm? Epidemiologists have debated for sixty years. Theories abound, but nobody knows. Perhaps concomitant bacterial or other infection played a major role, perhaps the stress of war or other environmental factors made a difference.

If so, well and good, for the times have changed and today we have potent antibiotics. But conceivably a large part of that pandemic mortality was due to some intrinsic feature of the virus, a characteristic that may be harbored even today on a gene fragment somewhere in the animal kingdom, a gene that could just possibly combine with human virus.

Despite impressions left by the swine flu affair, this remains a possibility. Ford could not accurately predict the killer and was thus severely limited in seeking to guard everyone against it. Mathews, Cooper and Sencer could not do so either. Neither could their scientific advisers. Nor can anyone in 1978. Only research, perhaps, someday will manage that.

APPENDICES

A

CAST OF

CHARACTERS

Persons named in chapters and in the chronology are identified by positions held when they first appear; if changes of position matter to the narration, these too are noted. Mindful of readers we tried in those chapters to minimize personal references, lest we present the reading problems of a Russian novel. Acknowledging that we have not wholly succeeded, we offer this list. It does not include Gerald R. Ford or Jimmy Carter. Otherwise we have endeavored to be complete. The list is alphabetical.

E. RUSSELL ALEXANDER, M.D., Member of Advisory Committee on Immunization Practices; Professor of Public Health, University of Washington.

ST. JOHN BARRETT, Deputy General Counsel of HEW, Ford Administration, to January 1977.

JOSEPH BARTLEY, M.D., Colonel and Chief of Preventive Medicine, Fort Dix.

RICHARD I. BEATTIE, Deputy General Counsel of HEW, Carter Administration, from January 1977.

PHILIP BRACHMAN, M.D., Director, Bureau of Epidemiology, Center for Disease Control.

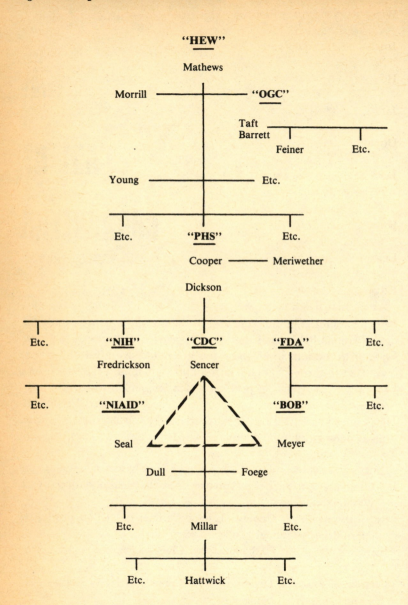

Selected Organizational Relationships in HEW, 1976
(includes individuals named in text)

WENDELL BRADFORD, Associate Director, Bureau of State Services, Center for Disease Control.

JOSEPH A. CALIFANO, JR., Secretary of HEW, Carter Administration, since January 1977.

HOWARD "BO" CALLAWAY, Campaign manager for President Ford to March 1976.

JAMES CANNON, Director of Domestic Council, Executive Office of the President, Ford Administration, to January 1977.

DONALD CARMODY, Director, Division of Health Protection, Office of Policy Development and Planning, Public Health Service.

JAMES CAVANAUGH, Deputy Chief of Staff in the White House and Deputy Director of the Domestic Council, Ford Administration, to January 1977.

HALE CHAMPION, Undersecretary of HEW, Carter Administration, from January 1977.

LESLIE CHEEK, Chief of Washington branch office, American Insurance Association.

RICHARD B. CHENEY, White House Chief of Staff, Ford Administration, to January 1977.

JOHN COCHRAN, White House Correspondent, National Broadcasting Company, to Winter 1977.

CHARLES COCKBURN, M.D., World Health Organization, Geneva, Switzerland.

LYLE CONRAD, Assistant Director, Immunization Division, Center for Disease Control.

JAMES COOPER, M.D., Special Assistant, Office of the Assistant Secretary for Health, Public Health Service.

THEODORE COOPER, M.D., Assistant Secretary for Health, HEW, Ford Administration, to January 1977.

JAMES F. DICKSON III, M.D., Deputy Assistant Secretary for Health under Cooper, Acting Assistant Secretary to June 1977.

LINDA DONALDSON, Staff attorney, Office of General Counsel, HEW, from Summer 1977.

WALTER R. DOWDLE, M.D., Director, Virology Division at Center for Disease Control.

H. BRUCE DULL, M.D., Assistant Director for Programs, Center for Disease Control.

CHARLES EDWARDS, M.D., Assistant Secretary for Health, HEW, Nixon Administration, to 1971.

BERNARD FEINER, Chief of Business and Administrative Law Division, Office of General Counsel, HEW.

JONATHAN E. FIELDING, M.D., Commissioner of Public Health, Commonwealth of Massachusetts.

ROBERT H. FINCH, Secretary of HEW, Nixon Administration, 1969–70.

DANIEL J. FLOOD, U.S. Representative from Pennsylvania, Chairman, Appropriations Subcommittee on Labor-HEW, House of Representatives.

WILLIAM H. FOEGE, M.D., Assistant Director for Operations, Center for Disease Control to April 1977; thereafter Director.

DONALD S. FREDRICKSON, M.D., Director, National Institutes of Health; reappointed, February 1977.

MAX L. FRIEDERSDORF, Assistant to the President for Legislative Affairs, Ford Administration, to January 1977.

JAMES GAITHER, Chairman of HEW Ethics Advisory Board from Spring 1977.

JOHN W. GARDNER, Secretary of HEW, Johnson Administration, 1965–67.

E. BURKE GIBLIN, Chairman of the Board, Parke-Davis Company, Detroit drug manufacturer.

MARTIN GOLDFIELD, M.D., Assistant Commissioner and chief Epidemiologist, Department of Public Health, New Jersey; relieved of these duties in 1977.

DAVID HAMBURG, M.D. Director, Institute of Medicine, National Academy of Sciences, to 1981.

MICHAEL HATTWICK, M.D., Chief of Respiratory and Special Pathogens Branch, Viral Disease Division, Bureau of Epidemiology, Center for Disease Control.

BEN W. HEINEMAN, JR., Executive Assistant to HEW Secretary Califano, from January 1977.

MAURICE R. HILLEMAN, Director, Virus and Cell Biological Research and Vice President, Merck, Sharpe & Dohme Research Laboratories.

JOHN J. HORAN, President, Merck & Company, Rahway, New Jersey (parent company of drug manufacturer).

LAWRENCE HOROWITZ, M.D., Consultant to (Kennedy) Subcommittee on Health, U.S. Senate.

LEE HYDE, M.D., Professional staff member, (Rogers) Subcommittee on Health and Environment, House of Representatives.

SPENCER JOHNSON, Associate Director, Domestic Council, Executive Office of the President, Ford Administration, to January 1977.

T. LAWRENCE JONES, Director, American Insurance Association, New York.

ALAN KENDAL, M.D., Virology Division, Center for Disease Control.

EDWARD M. KENNEDY, U.S. Senator from Massachusetts; Chairman, Senate Subcommittee on Health.

EDWIN D. KILBOURNE, M.D., Chairman, Department of Microbiology, Mt. Sinai School of Medicine, New York.

JOHN KNOWLES, M.D., President, Rockefeller Foundation, New York.

JOYCE C. LASHOF, M.D., Deputy Assistant Secretary for Health under Richmond to May 1978.

LOUISE L. LIANG, M.D., Special Assistant to the Secretary, HEW, from September 1977.

JAMES T. LYNN, Director, Office of Management and Budget, Executive Office of the President, Ford Administration, to January 1977.

WARREN G. MAGNUSON, U.S. Senator from Washington state, Chairman, Senate Appropriations Subcommittee on Labor-HEW.

ANDREW MAGUIRE, U.S. Representative from New Jersey; member, House Health Subcommittee.

DAVID MATHEWS, Secretary of HEW, Ford Administration, to January 1977.

MICHAEL McGINNIS, M.D., Special Assistant to HEW Secretary Califano; thereafter Deputy Assistant Secretary for Health.

JAMES McMANUS, Correspondent, Columbia Broadcasting System.

W. DELANO MERIWETHER, M.D., Special Assistant to Assistant Secretary for Health; Director, National Influenza Immunization Program, HEW.

HARRY M. MEYER, JR., M.D., Director, Bureau of Biologics, Food and Drug Administration.

ROBERT H. MICHEL, U.S. Representative from Illinois, Ranking Minority Member, Appropriations Subcommittee on Labor-HEW, House of Representatives.

J. DONALD MILLAR, M.D., Director, Bureau of State Services, Center for Disease Control.

WILLIAM MORRILL, Assistant Secretary for Planning and Evaluation, HEW, to January 1977.

J. ANTHONY MORRIS, Bacteriologist, Bureau of Biologics, Food and

Drug Administration; discharged under protest, July 1976.

DAVID NEWBERRY, Bureau of State Services, Center for Disease Control, on detail to National Influenza Immunization Program, Washington (Meriwether).

GARY NOBLE, M.D., Virology Division, Center for Disease Control.

PAUL O'NEILL, Deputy Director, Office of Management and Budget, Executive Office of the President, Ford Administration, to January, 1977.

THOMAS P. O'NEILL, U.S. Representative from Massachusetts, Majority Leader of the House of Representatives.

DENTON R. PETERSON, Immunization Program Representative, Minnesota State Health Department.

NEIL PETERSON, Chief, Torts Section, Civil Division, Department of Justice.

ROBERT C. PIERPOINT, White House Correspondent, Columbia Broadcasting System.

ELLIOT RICHARDSON, Secretary of HEW, Nixon Administration, to December 1972.

JULIUS B. RICHMOND, M.D., Assistant Secretary for Health, HEW, Carter Administration, from July 1977.

NELSON A. ROCKEFELLER, Vice President of the United States, Ford Administration, to January 1977.

PAUL G. ROGERS, U.S. Representative from Florida; Chairman, House Subcommittee on Health and the Environment.

WILLIAM P. ROGERS, Esq., Partner, Rogers and Wells, Washington, counsel to Richardson-Merrell (parent company of drug manufacturer).

DAVID K. ROWE, Director, Procurement and Grants Office, Center for Disease Control.

PHILIP RUSSELL, M.D., Colonel, Walter Reed Army Institute of Research.

ALBERT B. SABIN, M.D., Distinguished Research Professor of Biomedicine, Medical University, Charleston, S.C.

JONAS E. SALK, M.D., Founding Director, Salk Institute, San Diego, CA.

HAROLD SCHMECK, Medical reporter for the *New York Times*.

HARRY SCHWARTZ, Member, Editorial Board, *New York Times*.

JOHN R. SEAL, M.D., Scientific Director, National Institute for Allergy and Infectious Diseases (NIAID), National Institutes of Health, Public Health Service.

DAVID J. SENCER, M.D., Director, Center for Disease Control, to April 1977.

EILEEN SHANAHAN, Assistant Secretary for Public Affairs, HEW, Carter Administration, from January, 1977.

CAROLE SIMPSON, Correspondent, National Broadcasting Company.

REUEL A. STALLONES, M.D., Member, Advisory Committee on Immunization Practices; Dean, School of Public Health, University of Texas.

C. JOSEPH STETLER, President, Pharmaceutical Manufacturers Association, Washington.

WILLIAM HOWARD TAFT IV, General Counsel of HEW, Ford Administration, to January 1977.

STANLEY TEMKO, Esq., Partner, Covington and Burling, Washington, Counsel to Merck & Company (parent of Merck, Sharpe & Dohme, drug manufacturer).

FRANKLIN H. TOP, M.D., Colonel, Walter Reed Army Institute of Research.

HENRY A. WAXMAN, U.S. Representative from California; member, House Health Subcommittee.

CYRIL WECHT, M.D., County Coroner for Allegheny County (Pittsburgh) Health Department, Pennsylvania.

SIDNEY WOLFE, M.D., Director, Public Citizens Health Research Group (a Ralph Nader organization in Washington).

JOHN D. YOUNG, Assistant Secretary and Comptroller, HEW, Ford and Carter Administrations, through 1977.

VICTOR ZAFRA, Division chief, Office of Management and Budget.

B

TERMS AND

ORGANIZATIONS

Abbreviations

The shorthand references used throughout this study are identified as follows (listed alphabetically):

ACIP: Advisory Committee on Immunization Practices of the Public Health Service (in practice, of CDC).

AFEB: Armed Forces Epidemiological Board, Department of Defense.

AIA: American Insurance Association (casualty insurers), New York, Washington, D.C. and elsewhere.

AMA: American Medical Association.

BoB: The Bureau of Biologics in the Food and Drug Administration, an agency of the Public Health Service (not to be confused with the initials of the former name for the Office of Management and Budget).

CDC: Center for Disease Control, Atlanta, Ga., an agency of the Public Health Service.

DoD: U.S. Department of Defense.

GAO: U.S. General Accounting Office, an agency of Congress.

HEW: U.S. Department of Health, Education and Welfare.

HUD: U.S. Department of Housing and Urban Development.

NASA: National Aeronautics and Space Administration.

NCHS: National Center for Health Statistics, a unit of the Health Resources Administration in PHS.

NIAID: National Institute for Allergy and Infectious Diseases, Bethesda, Md., a unit of the National Institutes of Health in HEW.

NIH: National Institutes of Health, Bethesda, Md., an agency of the Public Health Service in HEW.

OGC: Office of General Counsel in the Department of Health, Education and Welfare.

OMB: Office of Management and Budget, a key agency in the Executive Office of the President.

OSTP: Office of Science and Technology Policy, a new agency in the Executive Office of the President; abolished (under a slightly different name) in 1969, revived in the Fall of 1976.

PERT: Program evaluation review technique. (Originally for weapons-systems.)

PHS: Public Health Service, a major administrative division of the Department of Health, Education and Welfare (not to be confused with the commissioned corps of the same name which staffs many positions but by no means all in that division).

PMA: Pharmaceutical Manufacturers Association, Washington, D.C.

R&D: Research and Development.

VA: Veterans Administration.

WHO: World Health Organization, Geneva, Switzerland.

SWINE FLU CHRONOLOGY

January 1976—March 1977

JANUARY 1976

5–Dr. Bruce Dull, Assistant Director for Programs of the Center for Disease Control (CDC), submits a memo to HEW Secretary David Mathews, sent via CDC director Dr. David Sencer and Assistant HEW Secretary for Health, Dr. Theodore Cooper; Dull states that liability problems may drive vaccine manufacturers out of business, and recommends that the Secretary support legislation to indemnify the manufacturers or to compensate all victims of vaccine

mid-January–large number of cases of respiratory disease are reported among Army recruits at Fort Dix, New Jersey; Walter Reed Army Laboratory identifies adenovirus as cause of earlier outbreak of respiratory disease at Fort Meade, Md.

22–Donald Carmody, a staff officer for Cooper in the Public Health Service, writes memo to his superior in the Office of Policy Development and Planning, emphasizing the problems in the Dull proposal and suggesting that it be sent up to Cooper without recommendation

27–Colonel Joseph Bartley, chief of preventive medicine at Fort Dix, reports outbreak of illness, presumed due to adenovirus, to local health department

28–Dr. Martin Goldfield, director of the New Jersey Public Health labs, contacts Bartley, gets briefing on the outbreak of respiratory disease, suspects influenza, and requests that throat washings be sent to the New Jersey state labs

29–eight throat washings from Fort Dix delivered to virus lab at N.J. Health Department

30–11 additional specimens from Fort Dix delivered to N.J. lab

FEBRUARY 1976

3–at the N.J. lab, 11 isolates are made from the 19 throat washings sent by Bartley from Fort Dix; most of these are identifiable as A Victoria or A Port Chalmers virus, but scientists are unable to identify two of the isolates and unsure about five others, so Goldfield sends these seven on to CDC and calls CDC's Dr. Gary Noble to report his findings

4–after leaving his sick bed and making a forced, five-mile, night march, Private David Lewis, Fort Dix recruit, collapses and dies

5–the 7 isolates mailed from New Jersey lab arrive at CDC's Bureau of Laboratories

5–CDC confirms that five of the seven New Jersey isolates are A Victoria; and other two appear to be influenza but do not type as A Victoria

10–the New Jersey lab sends to CDC two more unidentifiable isolates from Fort Dix, one of them taken from the deceased Lewis; N.J. lab finds soluble influenza A antigen in one unidentified isolate

11–CDC receives the second group of isolates

12–double immunodiffusion confirms two original untyped viruses are a type of influenza A; hemagglutinin inhibition tests indicate four of the Fort Dix isolates contain swine flu type hemagglutinin; CDC lab communicates this finding to Sencer in the evening

12–Goldfield telephones virologist Dr. Edwin Kilbourne of Mt. Sinai Hospital in New York City with the news that he possesses a virus he cannot type; Kilbourne asks Goldfield to send him some specimens

13–N.J. lab mails quantity of the Fort Dix virus to Kilbourne

13–scientists at CDC confirm that the isolates are indeed swine-type influenza A viruses; at Sencer's request, Dr. Walter Dowdle, head of CDC's labs, notifies scientists and health officials across the country of the A swine discovery, and invites them to a meeting at CDC the next day

14–emergency meeting is held at CDC to discuss the Fort Dix finding; in attendance are representatives of the Army (Dr. Philip Russell, Dr. Frank Top), the New Jersey Department of Health (Goldfield), FDA's Bureau of Biologics (Dr. Harry Meyer, Jr.), NIH's National Institute of Allergy and Infectious Diseases (Dr. John Seal), and CDC (Sencer–chairman, Dull, Dr. William Foege, Noble, Dr. Michael Hattwick, Dowdle, Dr. Alan Kendal); conferees discuss need to develop vaccine; also decide not to publicize swine virus finding

14–16–CDC reconfirms isolation and identification of swine flu virus from original throat swabs brought from N.J. Health Dept.

16–Sencer and Dowdle inform Dr. Charles Cockburn of the World Health Organization (Geneva) of swine virus finding; Dowdle informs Kilbourne

17–Kilbourne receives samples of the virus mailed from New Jersey; his lab begins to develop a fast-growing "recombinant" for use in vaccine

18–CDC notifies state health officials of swine flu finding

19–CDC calls press conference; Dull announces swine virus has been discovered at Fort Dix; makes no reference to the 1918 pandemic in his prepared remarks, but does in response to questions from reporters

20–first media coverage of swine flu focuses on CDC's announcement of the previous day; coverage links the Fort Dix virus to the 1918 pandemic

20–BoB hosts open workshop in Bethesda, Maryland, with representatives from the Armed Forces Epidemiological Board (AFEB), NIAID, CDC, the press, the scientific community, and all four vaccine-manufacturing companies; conferees discuss preparations for a swine flu immunization campaign; second meeting held in the afternoon to discuss surveillance plans

20–quantities of Fort Dix virus delivered to vaccine manufacturers, but virus grows poorly in their labs; companies await Kilbourne's recombined strain and some work on preparing their own

20–26–CDC alerts state epidemiologists in nationwide search for other cases of swine flu; besides earlier cases in Minnesota and Wisconsin, already known to CDC, the investigation turns up other isolated occurrences in Pennsylvania, Virginia, and Mississippi, although all but a questionable Virginia case involved human-pig contact

27–informal meetings are held at BoB; Sencer, Dowdle, Meyer, Seal, and Noble review status of swine flu investigation and discuss candidates for vaccine strain

MARCH 1976

1–9–Army conducts serosurveys at Fort Dix while CDC does the same in surrounding civilian populations; Army estimates as many as 500 recruits at Fort Dix may have been exposed to swine virus

9–as a prelude to the next day's meeting the Advisory Committee on Immunization Practices (ACIP), Sencer meets

Dowdle, Dull, Foege, and other staff from CDC's Epidemiology Bureau for an informal discussion regarding options; stockpiling of vaccine is discussed at some length

10–at an open meeting in Atlanta, CDC briefs the ACIP on the results of its preliminary investigations; ACIP members concur in need for major action, support production of vaccine and formulation of a plan to administer; stockpiling option is briefly mentioned; afterwards, Sencer telephones Cooper in Washington and summarizes meeting

12–AFEB holds meeting at Walter Reed Army Institute of Research to determine vaccine formulation for the military; Board recommends that swine component be incorporated into trivalent vaccine, along with A Victoria and B Hong Kong

13–Sencer finishes action-memorandum which he had prepared in the previous two days; memo calls for mass immunization campaign aimed at vaccinating all Americans, and recommends that Administration ask Congress for $134 million appropriation; proposes plan with Federal Government buying and testing the vaccine and setting dosage levels, the states distributing the vaccine, and public health agencies and private physicians administering it

13–Sencer asks Dr. Donald Millar, director of CDC's Bureau of State Services, to form a Program Implementation Group

13–Cooper leaves for eight-day trip to Egypt, with Acting Assistant Secretary James Dickson tending to affairs in his absence

15–At Secretary's morning staff meeting, Dickson, briefed by Sencer, summarizes swine flu problem

15–Dickson, Sencer and Meyer meet with Mathews for further discussion of problem; Sencer recommends mass immunization

15–Mathews sends brief note to James Lynn, Director of the Office of Management and Budget (OMB), informing him of the threat of a major flu epidemic; mentions that a supplementary appropriation may be needed in near future; requests the presence of OMB representatives at an afternoon meeting in his office

15–Sencer, Meyer and Seal brief Victor Zafra and assistants from OMB

15–President Gerald R. Ford first hears of the swine flu program from Lynn and Paul O'Neill, deputy director of OMB, along with James Cavanaugh, deputy director of the Domestic Council, in afternoon meetings on other subjects

17–18–Sencer telephones ACIP members to advise them of program specifics as set forth in his action-memorandum; invites their comments and gets unanimous assent

21–Cooper returns from Egypt

22–President meets with Mathews, Cooper and Dickson from HEW, Lynn and O'Neill from OMB, and Cavanaugh, James Cannon, Richard Cheney and Spencer Johnson from the White House to discuss swine virus finding; mass vaccination program is recommended to the President, but he postpones decision until he meets with leading scientists; schedules meeting for Wednesday, the 24th

24–President meets at White House with "blue-ribbon" panel of experts, including Dr. Jonas Salk, Dr. Albert Sabin, Dr. Fred Davenport, Kilbourne, Dr. Reuel Stallones, Sencer, and Meyer; following meeting, President goes before television cameras to announce that he is recommending a mass vaccination program for all Americans and urges that Congress immediately pass a special $135 million appropriation; afterwards, Mathews and Cooper conduct press conference

24–CDC initiates work on a "PERT" chart, plotting out steps and relationships in the swine flu program

25–Mathews sends memo to Cooper suggesting that he chair a coordinating Task Force for the "National Influenza Immunization Program"

25–BoB hosts open workshop in Bethesda; conferees include HEW officials, scientists from CDC, NIAID, Department of

Defense (DoD), and Veterans Administration (VA), university investigators, and drug company representatives, among others; group reviews developments relevant to program; vaccine trials discussed

30–hearing is held before the House Appropriations Subcommittee on Labor–Health, Education and Welfare (Rep. Daniel J. Flood, chairman); drug company spokesman, C. Joseph Stetler, talks of impending liability troubles and recommends government indemnification of vaccine manufacturers; subcommittee unanimously approves special appropriations (HJ Res 890)

31–hearing conducted before House Interstate and Foreign Commerce Subcommittee on Health and the Environment (Rep. Paul G. Rogers, chairman); need for authorization bill discussed

31–White House sends memo to all Federal departments and agencies, requesting support for the immunization program

APRIL 1976

1–Senate Labor and Public Welfare Subcommittee on Health (Sen. Edward M. Kennedy, chairman) holds hearings on swine flu program; Kennedy presses hard on lagging immunization rates for childhood diseases

2–CDC conducts large meeting in Atlanta with state health officers and representatives of private medicine to explain proposed swine flu program; Sencer outlines desired state participation; state officials question CDC hard on funding of local programs; Goldfield challenges wisdom of decision to mass immunize; TV Evening News broadcasts his dissent

2–House Appropriations Committee reports out special appropriations bill (HJ Res 890) containing $135 million for swine flu program

5–Richard Friedman, HEW Regional Director (Chicago), sends memo to Cooper in which he suggests that PHS seriously consider stockpiling, avoid "scare tactics," and provide more financial support for state programs

5–Rogers subcommittee approves authorization bill (HR 13012); in the press for time, bill is not sent to full Commerce Committee, but directly to the House floor

5–House approves authorization bill by voice vote, and then, after limited debate, approves appropriations resolution, 354–12

5–in a letter to the Pharmaceutical Manufacturers Association (PMA) Cooper says that the manufacturers' concern over liability should be alleviated by the Federal Government's assuming the duty to warn

6–Senate Appropriations Committee (Sen. Warren Magnuson, chairman) conducts a hearing on the special appropriation

7–Veterans Administration gives CDC the authority to negotiate and administer vaccine contracts for VA staff and patients; requests 1.5 million doses

7–8–WHO holds meeting in Geneva with consultants from 15 countries; conferees discuss implications of swine outbreak and recommend that worldwide surveillance be increased, that poorer nations devise contingency plans, and that countries with production capability decide for themselves whether or not to produce swine vaccine

8–Senate Appropriations Committee approves HJ Res 890 and reports it out, after adding $1.8 billion of job support funds; Committee Report indicates that no Federal agency is to assume liability which it had not assumed for previous immunization programs; PMA telegrams a protest to the President

8–An unidentified senior official of the Federal Insurance Company (Chubb Corporation) advises corporate headquarters of Merck, the parent company of Merck, Sharpe & Dohme (one of the vaccine manufacturers), that effective July 1 it will exclude from Merck's product liability coverage all indemnity and defense costs associated with claims arising out of the swine flu program

9–Senate Labor and Public Welfare Committee does not act on the House authorization bill (HR 13012), nor does it pass an authorization measure of its own; after a minor floor amendment is added, the full Senate approves the appropriations bill, 61–7

9–Cooper announces Dr. W. Delano Meriwether as director of the National Influenza Immunization Program

9–Meyer sends memo to Cooper in which he estimates production timetable for vaccine; says manufacturers will begin to produce in June and should be able to turn out 24–30 million doses per month, provided they are able to get 2 doses per egg

12–House passes the amended appropriations bill by voice vote; thus, no authorization bill is passed, and appropriation is made under Title III of the Public Health Service Act. Colloquies on the Senate floor and a statement on the House floor by Congressman Robert H. Michel of Illinois tend to negate effect of the language on liability in Senate Committee report

12–Cavanaugh chairs a White House meeting on the swine flu program

12–T. Lawrence Jones, president of the American Insurance Association (casualty insurers), meets with Lynn of OMB; at end of session, Jones mentions that the insurance industry will not insure the manufacturers for swine vaccine unless the Government extends further liability protection

13–the President and Chairman of Merck writes to Secretary Mathews, copies to White House and CDC, among others, stressing that liability will become a critical problem if the drug companies do not receive additional protection; emphasis is on duty-to-warn; warning from insurers is included but not headlined

14–CDC issues to the states its "Immunization Program Guidelines for Grant Applications"

14–HEW Office of General Counsel (OGC) holds first meeting with Washington counsel to the drug manufacturers; antitrust and liability problems are discussed, particularly the Federal Government's assumption of the duty to warn

15–President signs the special appropriations bill into law (PL 94–266)

15–NIAID hosts workshop in Bethesda to discuss plans for flu vaccine trials

20–Cavanaugh chairs another meeting at the White House on the progress of immunization plans

21–press conference is held at HEW to announce the beginning of vaccine field trials; 3000 volunteers are to be involved

27–CDC completes its PERT chart

30–HEW Press Analysis tracks news coverage from 111 newspapers in 60 cities; shows that editorial response to the swine flu program in April has been 88 percent favorable

MAY 1976

1–other manufacturers of swine flu vaccine (Merrell, Parke-Davis, Wyeth) receive notice from casualty insurers about cancellation of liability coverage for swine vaccine

5–at a meeting between OGC negotiators and attorneys for the drug companies, Stanley Temko, counsel to Merck, urges Administration to press for legislation which would indemnify the manufacturers for all costs not directly tied to their own negligence in production

6–St. John Barrett of OGC sends memo to Cooper setting forth bargaining positions of OGC and the manufacturers; advises against the Federal Government's doing more than assuming the duty to warn

6–Cooper sends letter to selected newspapers, explaining the swine flu program and urging favorable public response

6–7–ACIP meets in Atlanta to review progress of program; committee agrees that full preparations should continue, although Dr. Russell Alexander suggests that the final decision to vaccinate might be postponed pending further swine flu outbreak; consensus still opposes stockpiling, however; committee also approves risk-benefit statement for use in Vaccinee Consent Form

14–information packet mailed to Immunization Project directors in states

15–CDC asks state health officials to contribute to development of informed consent procedures

17–in an address delivered at the College of Pharmacy at the University of Toledo, Sabin suggests that the vaccine ought to be stockpiled pending a new outbreak

18–CDC signs a contract for the purchase of 1400–2000 jet injectors

19–first technical meeting at BoB with manufacturers regarding production of vaccine

21,24–meeting held between Washington counsel to the manufacturers and OGC negotiators, including General Counsel William Howard Taft IV; William P. Rogers, representing Merrell, informs OGC that Merrell will not participate unless it is assured of complete indemnity for those functions assumed by the Government

24–Mathews delegates authority to CDC to award flu grants to states

25–OGC memo to Mathews through Cooper traces difficulty with manufacturers over liability issue; sets forth contract clause representing maximum Government concession within existing law; mentions Merrell's refusal to proceed without indemnification

26–conference of State and Territorial Health Epidemiologists is held at Cherry Hill, N.J.; immunization program is discussed

27–CDC issues requests to the four manufacturers for "Vaccine Production Proposals," to be submitted by June 15;

cover letter sets goal of initial deliveries in July, with all 40 million bivalent doses delivered by September 1, 120 of the 160 million monovalent doses delivered by September 1, and the rest of the monovalent by November 15

27–HEW begins to prepare legislation authorizing indemnification of the manufacturers against all claims other than those based on negligence

27–CDC representatives (Foege, Wendell Bradford) consult with DoD on vaccine for the armed forces

28–in a conference call with Cooper, Sencer and Seal, Meyer estimates that 196 million doses of vaccine will be available by November 1

31–HEW Press Analysis for May shows a slight drop-off in the amount of coverage for the swine flu program; indicates that editorial approval of the program has waned, from 88 percent favorable to 66 percent favorable

JUNE 1976

2–Cooper announces that Parke-Davis used the wrong virus in the manufacture of 2 million doses; implies that this alone may result in 4–6 week delay for the start of vaccinations

2–second technical meeting at BoB with manufacturers regarding production of the vaccine; Meyer estimates that 288 million doses could be available by January 1, 1977

2–Cooper sends memo through Mathews' office to the White House stating that legislation would be needed to secure Merrell's participation, which is necessary to program

8–DoD makes known to CDC its preferred dosage specifications for monovalent and bivalent vaccine (600 CCA swine, 400 CCA Victoria)

10–casualty insurer tells Parke-Davis that as of July 1 it will not be covered for swine vaccine; Merrell receives same message from its new insurer shortly after

11–CDC mails "Weekend Flu Facts" to state health officers, informing them of continuing liability issues and denouncing editorial position of *New York Times*

14–Parke-Davis executive writes to Cooper, warns that his company may lose insurance coverage on July 1 if not fully relieved of liability for vaccine damage; states unwillingness of Parke-Davis to self-insure

15–E. Burke Giblin, Chairman of the Board of Parke-Davis, sends telegram to the President, Congress and other Federal officials, detailing the July 1 insurance cut-off and requesting legislative assistance

15–Cooper announces that Administration will ask Congress to pass indemnification legislation

15–25–manufacturers submit first production proposals, which suggest that only 80 million doses can be delivered by October 1, 146 million by December 1, with first shipments to be made in July

16–Administration submits proposals to Congress (HR 14409) authorizing HEW to indemnify the manufacturers against damages attributed to swine flu vaccination, except for those claims involving charges of negligent manufacture or breach of contract

16–CBS Evening News reports the manufacturers have given the Government notice that they will no longer be insured for production of swine vaccine as of July 1, and that the insurers are reluctant to extend such coverage because "they fear the costs involved in defending against claims resulting from unforeseen side effects"

17–third technical meeting at BoB between manufacturers and virologists from CDC and BoB

18–CDC issues Supplemental Guidelines for Influenza Immunization Project Grants, dealing specifically with informed consent problem; CDC also releases statement of risks and benefits for the informed consent form

21–NIAID hosts meeting in Bethesda to review the results of field trials; results indicate that adults can be safely and effectively vaccinated with a 200 CCA dose of the swine vaccine, but that no acceptable dose has been found for young adults and children

22–as a follow-up to the previous day, the ACIP meets in Bethesda with the BoB's Advisory Panel on Viral and Rickettsial Vaccines to make dosage recommendations; group recommends 200 CCA dose of monovalent for those over 25 (bivalent for those over 65 and others in high-risk group); further tests will be needed before recommendations can be made for the sub-18 or 18–24 age groups

24–meeting at CDC, with Sencer, Dowdle, and others, to review production schedules submitted by manufacturers

25–casualty spokesman, Leslie Cheek, Washington representative of AIA, places conference telephone call to Meriwether, Meyer, Sencer, and other CDC officials; announces that none of the manufacturers will be insured after July 1, and that, as matters stand, the drug companies will not be able to find insurance anywhere

28–the Rogers subcommittee conducts hearing on the Administration's indemnification bill; committee members are unsympathetic to the proposal, Administration witnesses are lukewarm in their advocacy, and insurance spokesman Cheek is questioned hard

30–HEW Press Analysis for June indicates that coverage of program in major newspapers has dropped some from May levels, but that percentage of favorable reports remains at two-thirds

JULY 1976

1–non-profit health group convenes a swine flu forum in New York City; Dull speaks, and says that parallels with 1918 are inappropriate, that there is no reason to fear that a 1976 epidemic would equal the 1918 pandemic in scale

1–the Rogers subcommittee holds an informal session with drug company executives to analyze the lack of progress on the liability issue; subsequently, the subcommittee tables the Administration's indemnification bill, and Chairman Rogers tells HEW General Counsel Taft to reach a contractual solution with the manufacturers and insurers that will not require new legislation

2–manufacturers meet with officials from the Justice Dept. and OGC to discuss possible contractual solutions; no progress is made, and Cooper subsequently releases press statement explaining the impasse

5–7–OGC and the manufacturers agree on contract language, but manufacturers refuse to sign unless Justice Dept. officials approve the language; also, the manufacturers indicate that they will wait on the response of their insurers, to be forthcoming by July 13

7–Cooper receives "Program Overview" from OGC outlining state and local liability problems

8–HEW asks Justice Dept. for opinion on proposed contract language

9–insurance representatives meet with the manufacturers to discuss the proposed language, and agree that it is not sufficient

9–after meeting with the President, Mathews announces that he personally has offered to mediate between manufacturers and insurers, and has scheduled a meeting for the 13th

9–Dull writes ACIP members, explaining problems in the determination of vaccine dosage levels for children, and setting forth possible solutions for their consideration

11–Justice Dept. tells Taft that the proposed contract language would not violate the Anti-Deficiency Act

12–after three years of proceedings the FDA Administrator dismisses Dr. J. Anthony Morris, a researcher in BoB, charging insubordination and incompetent performance; Morris goes public, charging he is being punished for findings that cast doubt on safety of influenza vaccines and immunization

13–insurance company officials participate in OGC-drug company meetings for the first time; manufacturers indicate willingness to give contract language a try but insurers demur; Mathews holds press conference

13–Ad Hoc Committee of AFEB meets to discuss immunization program and vaccine composition for armed forces; afterwards, representatives of CDC and AFEB meet, and the latter request whole virus vaccine in 400 CCA doses; CDC defers final decision

13–CDC meets with labor organizations and large industries to disseminate information and solicit their support

14–staff meeting held at CDC with representatives of all PHS Regional Centers to discuss progress of state programs

15–Merrell verbally notifies Cooper it will not purchase eggs after Tuesday, July 20, thus ceasing vaccine production. Cooper also learns that Parke-Davis will decide within weeks on termination of its own production

15–CDC issues Revised Guidelines on Informed Consent, as well as Information Forms for monovalent and bivalent vaccine

16–19–HEW staffers following liability meet to consider options for solving problem; consideration given to dropping program, but consensus reached that White House should be used to break deadlock

18–31–CDC investigates reported outbreaks of swine flu elsewhere in the world, including Manila and Taiwan, but all leads are false

19–drug companies inform HEW that they are still unable to obtain insurance, and will soon have to cease manufacture

19–after meeting with Mathews, President Ford holds press conference and announces that Administration will find a way to carry out the immunization program "with or without the support of Congress"

19—Cooper sends memo to the White House, listing the program's problems and reviewing available options to deal with each; raises termination of program as one option, and limitation to high-risk group as another, but rejects both, and recommends continuation of mass immunization

20—Rogers subcommittee conducts another hearing on the liability problem, examining the progress of negotiations among OGC, the manufacturers and the insurers

20—CDC sends letter to state health departments urging continuation of plans to vaccinate entire population; letter contains ACIP's recommendations on dosages for the 18-to-24 age group

21—in response to White House query, the manufacturers explain their objections to "contract solution"; letters sent to Cooper, then forwarded to White House

21–23—CDC holds meetings at its Regional Offices with state health officers, Immunization Project Directors, and Public Health Advisors

22—American Insurance Association sends memo to Cooper; explains that the industry refuses to provide coverage because: (1) the legal climate is too unsettled to permit actuarial calculation, (2) the casualty insurance industry lost more than $7 billion worldwide underwriting product liability in 1974 and 1975, and (3) the insurers feel that the Federal Government ought to defend all claims

22–23—ACIP meets in Atlanta and recommends that program continue as planned

23—Rogers subcommittee continues hearings; insurance executives appear, and are widely assailed for non-support; one of them suggests an insurance pool, but the others are not receptive to the idea

23—President sends letter to Rogers urging that Congress pass indemnification legislation quickly

23,26–at the urging of Mathews, insurers formulate private insurance plans; insurers' discussions with OGC negotiators produce no solutions

27–insurers offer three private plans; OGC and the drug companies veto two of the proposals, but ask the insurers to obtain industry commitments for full participation in the third

30–insurers, manufacturers, and HEW officials meet to make final decision on private insurance program; insurers report failure to fully subscribe excess levels of plan; when pressured, three manufacturers promise to continue production in the immediate future, but Merrell, having already discontinued production, does not commit itself to resumption

30–Mathews tells Rogers about the private insurance impasse and says legislation is needed

AUGUST 1976

2–outbreak of mysterious disease reported in Philadelphia; swine flu mentioned as possible cause of so-called Legionnaire's Disease

2–HEW and subcommittee staff draft new bill, introduced as HR 15050 and S 3735; measure is modeled on Tort Claims Act and stipulates that all claims arising from the program are to be filed with the Federal Government

2–after telephone calls to drug companies, Dowdle reports that 125 million doses are prepared in bulk

3–Rogers subcommittee conducts mark-up session of House bill; Mathews then speaks before subcommittee, and says that there is a "possibility" that swine flu is responsible for the Philadelphia deaths; subsequently, the subcommittee reports out HR 15050 by a 6–4 vote

5–House Commerce Committee considers the Tort Claims bill, but decides not to report it after receiving word that Legionnaire's Disease is *not* swine flu; committee postpones further action until August 10

5–Kennedy subcommittee conducts hearing on Senate bill, S 3735; Sencer testifies that the mystery disease is almost certainly not swine flu; but members express concern about possibility of link; subcommittee approves the measure

6–the President, alarmed by indications that congressional enthusiasm for the bill is waning, urges prompt passage before TV cameras; says he is "dumbfounded" by unwillingness of Congress to act

6–Senate adopts resolution discharging S 3735 from the Labor and Public Welfare Committee and sending the measure directly to the Senate floor

6–insurance executives begin to prepare an insurance program for the manufacturers which would extend $220 million coverage, excess of $10 million self-insured

7–8–staffs of interested legislators and government consultants work on the bill, inserting a number of favorite provisions

9–at a meeting of insurance company executives and brokers in Washington, the first layer of $20 million is quickly subscribed; 25 percent of the second layer is also taken; industry officials are confident that the balance of the second level will be subscribed

10–President telephones House Speaker Carl Albert and urges that the Tort Claims bill be reported to the House floor under a no-amendment rule

10–after reviewing S 3735, the Senate Appropriations Committee clears it for floor consideration, without endorsement

10–Rogers makes last-minute attempt to muster a quorum in the House Commerce Committee to report out the House version of the bill, but fails

10–House proponents of the bill work with Senate sponsors to redraft S 3735, incorporating changes suggested by the House Commerce and Judiciary Committees

10–by voice vote, Senate adopts the redrafted version of the Tort Claims bill; afterwards, the House approves the measure too, under a no-amendment rule

11–representatives of HEW and the drug companies meet for the fourth time at BoB to make arrangements for the distribution of vaccine

11–at a news conference, Meriwether announces the program is more than two months behind schedule and that immunization will start in late September; says all states and 13 cities and territories have developed and submitted plans for vaccination programs

12–President signs the Tort Claims bill into law, PL 94–380

12–manufacturers and HEW officials meet to work out final schedule of dosage levels for the vaccination of all those over 18

13–CDC telegrams vaccine manufacturers and asks them to submit revised proposals for vaccine delivery; accompanies request with two announcements: (1) CDC is reducing minimum guarantees for monovalent vaccine from 100 million to 50 million doses; (2) final delivery deadline has been set at December 3

15–contract is signed between CDC and Opinion Research Corporation to conduct monthly surveys of public attitudes toward program

17–meeting is held in Atlanta between CDC and members of the National Commission for the Protection of Human Subjects of Biomedical and Behavioral Research to determine the adequacy of informed consent forms; commission disapproves CDC's format, offers suggestions

18–OGC negotiators Taft and Bernard Feiner along with Sencer and David K. Rowe, director of CDC's Procurement and Grants office, meet with counsel to the manufacturers in order to arrive at an understanding of the effects of PL 94–380; agreement reached in all areas except "limitation on contractor profit"

19–fifth technical meeting is held at BoB with representatives of NIAID and OGC, as well as the drug companies, present

19–having received notice of the December 3 deadline, Parke-Davis advises CDC that it will cease initiating production of new batches on August 21 unless the delivery deadline is extended; Sencer telegrams back, asking Parke-Davis not to stop production but requesting at the same time that the company aim at the announced December 3 deadline

20–final draft for vaccine labelling is delivered by BoB to the manufacturers

20–representatives from the four companies meet at CDC to review basis for determining "cost" of production

20–24–manufacturers submit revised production estimates, promising 20 million doses by October 1, 193 million by December 3

28–OGC approves an Introductory Statement Concerning Influenza Vaccination and announces that the Statement will be appended to the informed consent form previously developed by CDC

30–Merrell is first company to submit batches of vaccine to BoB for testing

31–Mathews sends letter to all manufacturers, asking them to redouble efforts to produce more vaccine earlier

31–Parke-Davis telegrams to CDC, explaining that it would no longer initiate new production of vaccine as of September 2 unless the December deadline were extended

31–a Gallup Poll conducted in late August corroborates the results of a National Survey taken early in August; Poll shows 93 percent of Americans aware of immunization program (same as in National Survey), and 52 percent intend to get shot (vs. 53 percent in Survey)

SEPTEMBER 1976

1–HEW makes public the production estimates of the manufacturers, as revised in late August

1–HEW gives CDC authority to sign "letter" contracts with the manufacturers, until such time as cost and pricing methods could be negotiated for use in final contracts

2–President holds emergency meeting with Mathews, at which the Secretary guarantees that there will be enough vaccine to permit every American over age 18 who wishes to receive shot to do so by January or February

2–CDC responds to Parke-Davis telegram of August 31 by stating that the company should try to increase production before December 3, as urged by Mathews

2–BoB approves first batches of vaccine for release

3–manufacturers answer charges that they delayed production by claiming that they are operating at full capacity, and have been for months; Merrell says it stopped production of bulk only upon fulfillment of its initial quota

3–NIAID workshop is held in Bethesda to plan long-term surveillance of vaccine recipients

3–brokers for insurance companies write participating companies, detailing procedures for insuring manufacturers

8–Committee on Infectious Diseases of the American Academy of Pediatrics meets in Atlanta with officials from BoB, CDC, NIAID, and ACIP to make recommendation on vaccination of the 3-to-18 age group; committee recommends two doses of split virus, bivalent vaccine spaced four weeks apart, for high risk population only; committee declines to make recommendation for healthy youngsters, 3–18, pending further study

8–CDC sends all manufacturers a letter asking them to ship available vaccine prior to October 1, with assurances that it will not be used until October 1

8–Cooper instructs CDC to extend delivery date for vaccine to January 15

10–insurance company representatives inform House Health Subcommittee that the insurance program is fully subscribed

10—Sencer, Meyer, and Seal agree to schedule an open meeting on children's vaccination as soon as possible after October 15

13—Rogers subcommittee continues hearings; Administration officials admit that production is behind schedule, outline timetable for delivery of vaccine

13—Mathews issues final "cost" and "profit" criteria for vaccine contracts

13–22—letter contracts signed with all four vaccine manufacturers, stipulating that delivery deadline is to be extended to January 15

14—Jones of the American Insurance Association writes Mathews to suggest he convene a national conference of interested parties to discuss liability problem in government-sponsored public health campaigns

17—CDC issues revised Guidelines of Informed Consent, incorporating the "Introduction" approved by HEW on August 28

20—the president of the National Commission for the Protection of Human Subjects writes to Sencer, expressing some reservation about the incorporation of the "Introduction" into the previously prepared consent form; says it is a "good faith" effort, but still worrisome

22—letter contracts between manufacturers and CDC are completed; contracts contain the manufacturers' newly revised production estimates, which show further reduction in deliveries—only 109 million doses by December 1, 146 million by January 15

22—Merck makes first shipment of vaccine to states

23—Kennedy subcommittee conducts hearing on polio immunization and the need for a National Commission to set immunization policy; Dickson tells subcommittee that HEW will convene a National Immunization Conference to discuss long-range Federal immunization policy and draft recommendations

24–CDC issues Supplemental Project Grant Guidelines, dealing with: (1) steps to be taken to notify persons in the 18-to-24 age bracket of need for second shot; (2) reiteration of high risk definition; and (3) a prohibition against giving vaccination before October 1

29–CDC announces that immunization program will officially begin with vaccinations at the state fair in Indianapolis, Indiana

OCTOBER 1976

1–first swine flu shots given

1–Taft sends Cooper memo describing how contracts with vaccine manufacturers will include a fund to cover the $2.5 million self-insurance retained by each manufacturer

11–three elderly Pittsburgh people die shortly after receiving inoculation at same clinic

12–Pittsburgh health officials decide to close down the immunization program in Allegheny County pending investigation of the deaths; health officials in nine states follow suit, and six other program areas suspend use of vaccine drawn from the same batch as used in the Pittsburgh clinic

12–at a news conference in Atlanta, Sencer says CDC has sent epidemiologists to investigate, but that thus far there is no evidence to suggest the deaths were caused by vaccine

12–preliminary autopsy results are released on two of the three elderly persons whose deaths touched off the scare; results indicate that cause of death in each case was heart attack; however, Allegheny County Coroner Dr. Cyril Wecht sounds skeptical on the TV Evening News; suggests deaths may not have been coincidental

13–body count begins; Millar issues press release saying that 14 persons in 9 states reportedly died after receiving shot; says numbers are well within range of the expected for first two weeks of the program and that no evidence has been found linking any of the deaths with vaccine

13—BoB reports completed tests on the batch of vaccine used in the Pittsburgh clinic, with no finding of contamination

14—33 persons now reported as having died following vaccination

14—President and family receive shots before television cameras

14—Cooper holds news conference to summarize results of the investigation; says both vaccine and immunization program are exonerated, and decries "body count mentality"; all states which suspended either have resumed by now, or will soon; several areas report rapidly falling vaccination rate

14—on his network radio broadcast, Walter Cronkite chides news media for coverage of Pittsburgh deaths

21—Sencer writes to manufacturers, asking them to reassess production and delivery capabilities in light of extended deadline

22—meeting sponsored by NIAID at Bethesda to review latest vaccine trials with the 3-to-18 age group; Seal announces that persons in this group can be safely and effectively immunized with 2 doses of split virus vaccine administered four weeks apart; says such administration will not begin until formal recommendation is made by ACIP sometime in next few weeks

22—CDC announces 41 deceased vaccinees to date; still no known connection to vaccine

25—Leslie Cheek of the AIA writes Rogers, summarizing the insurers' underwriting of program

29—Sencer sends telegrams to states, explaining that final dosage recommendation for children is still pending

NOVEMBER 1976

4–10–CDC develops options for vaccinating children; also considers recommending second dose for the 18-to-24 age group

5–*New York Times* prints article by Sabin criticizing the handling of the swine flu program; says decision to proceed in March was justifiable, but the use of 1918 "scare tactics" was not; favors a stockpiling, preparedness approach

6–a National Survey is released, containing results of poll taken October 4–12; indicates that only 1 percent of eligible population had received shot by October 12, but another 57 percent intended to receive shot in future

6–alarmed by results of the October National Survey, which showed a particularly poor immunization rate in the black population, Cooper sends letters to managers of inner city radio stations, requesting support and providing sample copy for public service spots

12–Millar writes to states, informing them of invigorated "Awareness" campaign

12–case of Guillain-Barré syndrome in Minnesota vaccinee

12–14–National Immunization Conference organized by Cooper is held at the National Institutes of Health in Bethesda to draft national policy on immunization; six major issues are identified: (1) development of policy, (2) consent, (3) production and supply, (4) liability, (5) research and development, and (6) health information and public awareness; it is decided that work groups will be formed to study these issues and report back at a second conference in March or April 1977

15–ACIP recommends that healthy persons in the 3–18 age group be given two doses of split virus vaccine four weeks apart; also announces that only 8 million doses of such vaccine remain, and thus only 4 million of the 57 million persons in this category will be able to get shot; in addition,

ACIP recommends that a second dose be given to those in 18-to-24 age group

15–19–initial investigation by Minnesota Department of Health into occurrences of Guillain-Barré syndrome in vaccinees

17–Taft writes the Internal Revenue Service concerning the tax status of the manufacturers' self-insurance fund

18–Cooper expresses concern over the low level of participation nationwide; only four project areas over the 50 percent mark (Wyoming, Hawaii, Puerto Rico, and Trust Territories)

19–report is made of seroconversion to swine virus in 32-year-old man in Concordia, Missouri

21–*New York Times* poll shows that over half of those New York City residents who have not received shot feel it is unnecessary

22–Missouri state health officials confirm the swine flu case in Concordia

22–Parke-Davis submits official reply to the charge that it had negligently manufactured millions of doses of vaccine; in answer to HEW charge that it had carelessly used an A Shope strain instead of A swine, Parke-Davis claims total innocence, and suggests that CDC may have given it wrong strain at start

23–CDC epidemiologists report no evidence of human-to-human transmission of swine virus in Concordia

24–New York City, New Jersey and Connecticut all report increases in vaccination rate following swine finding in Missouri

24–Denton Peterson, Immunization Program Representative in the Minnesota Department of Health, calls CDC to discuss case of Guillain-Barré syndrome in vaccinee

DECEMBER 1976

2–Minnesota reports three additional cases of Guillain-Barré at same time as Alabama reports three cases; CDC begins investigation

3–isolate taken from a 23-year-old hog farmer in Wisconsin is identified as swine virus; subsequent search indicates sick swine the source and some secondary spread spotted

6–CDC ships Public Awareness materials to project directors, and to radio and television stations

7–CDC confirms that isolate taken from Wisconsin man is swine virus

9–Lyle Conrad, assistant director of the Immunization Division at CDC, announces that measles cases are up 64 percent nationwide from last year; blames the swine flu program, which he claims has diverted resources from more needy programs

11–investigation of Guillain-Barré is extended to eleven states

13–Sencer makes a conference call to outside experts; reports preliminary data on the association of Guillain-Barré with the vaccine, and seeks their opinions; consensus is that program should not be halted

14–CDC issues press release on Guillain-Barré; says that 54 cases in 10 states have thus far been reported, and of the 54, 30 received shot anywhere from one to thirty days before onset of symptoms

14–Dowdle prepares a reply to Parke-Davis on the matter of the mistaken production of Shope vaccine; refutes the contention of Parke-Davis that CDC was at fault, and reiterates that the company must be held to have been negligent and not paid for the faulty doses

15–Sencer makes second conference call regarding the Guillain-Barré problem

16–Sencer conducts morning conference call, his third in four days, with 20 experts from NIAID, BoB and the states, conferees agree on recommendation of a one-month suspension to allow for investigation of link; Sencer calls Cooper with the recommendation; Cooper confers with Mathews and Cavanaugh; telephones Salk; President okays suspension

16–subsequently, Sencer in Atlanta and Cooper in Washington announce suspension of the program

16–Rogers subcommittee conducts an emergency hearing to get explanation of moratorium from HEW officials

17–Kennedy subcommittee holds a hearing; chairman says program is dead, and Cooper agrees that it would be difficult to get program started again, if and when such is recommended; Foege estimates incidence of Guillain-Barré in vaccinated group is about four times greater than normal

17–Millar sends notice from CDC to all project areas explaining moratorium; Dr. Phil Brachman writes state epidemiologists, asking that they survey all Guillain-Barré reported after September 1

20–swine virus is isolated from 13-year-old boy in Wisconsin; subsequent investigation indicates pigs are source of infection

23–Cooper submits first of several weekly reports to Congress on the Guillain-Barré evidence

29–ACIP advises against resuming the program since several more weeks may be needed to investigate; recommends that shot should be available to individual patients if both doctor and patient agree that vaccine is needed and if patient is fully informed

30–HEW announces that the Federal Government has received a total of 31 claims valued at $1.2 million under the Tort Claims bill

30–in Vail, Colorado, President tells TV news reporters that he concurred in the December decision to suspend, but defends the original March decision to immunize everyone

late December–HEW fills out the membership of the six work groups created at the Immunization Conference in November; broad cross-section of interests represented; work groups asked to submit reports by March 1 and plan on an early April conference

JANUARY 1977

5–CBS Evening News airs a lengthy piece on the issue of declining immunization rates against childhood diseases

6–Cooper announces resignation, effective Inauguration Day

11–representatives of HEW and the Department of Justice meet to discuss procedure for handling claims filed under PL 94–380

11–Minnesota Health Department reports case of swine flu in a 27-year-old man who has had contact with pigs; no human-to-human transmission is discovered

11–Cooper asks Sencer and CDC for advice on reformulation of informed consent forms

14–ACIP meets in Atlanta and concludes that the moratorium on all influenza vaccine ought to be lifted; observes that flu shots do appear to entail some slight additional risk of contracting Guillain-Barré (estimated at one case for every 100,000 to 200,000 vaccinations); recommends that main focus of resumed program should be on high-risk group

14–subsequently, Sencer reads draft of recommendations over phone to Cooper, who concurs

16–Sencer releases final ACIP recommendations after double-checking with members by telephone; group recommendation is resumption on limited scale, aimed at high-risk group

17–in deference to incoming Administration, Cooper declines to decide whether or not to lift the moratorium

18–in response to Cooper's letter of January 11, Sencer sends memo to the Assistant Secretary setting forth the options for the future of the program, and strongly recommends that Cooper concur with the recommendation of the ACIP to resume on a limited scale

18–Cooper responds immediately to Sencer, asking that he: (1) poll the states on their willingness to rejoin the battle, (2) estimate the cost of restarting the program, and (3) develop a new informed consent form, and get the concurrence of OGC and the National Commission for the Protection of Human Subjects

18–CDC formulates new Informed Consent forms, incorporating a warning on the possibility of the vaccinee contracting Guillain-Barré

19–Sencer responds to Cooper, listing the results of CDC's poll of the states; few expressed themselves as willing to resume a full-scale public program; Sencer estimates that the start-up cost would be between $15,000 and $30,000; Sencer also sends Cooper the new Informed Consent forms

19–Cooper issues news release explaining his decision not to lift the moratorium; says that Informed Consent forms are still a problem, that the states must be consulted individually about scale of resumption, and that a proper scope and target had to be selected for revised program

20–Califano sworn in as Secretary of HEW

20–21–NIAID workshop on the vaccine test program is held in Bethesda; some criticism leveled on the limited amount of follow-up surveillance that is being done

25–BoB workshop is held in Bethesda; in attendance are representatives from CDC, NIAID, DoD, and manufacturing firms; conferees discuss alternatives for vaccine composition for 1977–1978

26–Acting Assistant Secretary for Health Dickson sends memo to Califano, sketching the history of the swine flu program and itemizing the major options for dealing with the current moratorium

28–OMB approves a Department of Justice supplemental budget of $1.2 million for swine flu litigation in 1977; Justice officials estimate that an equivalent appropriation will be needed for the same purpose through 1980

28–World Health Organization announces its 1977–1978 recommendation for influenza vaccine composition

FEBRUARY 1977

2–BoB prepares reply to Parke-Davis on the Shope vaccine matter, claiming that Parke-Davis was negligent and that it ought not to be paid

2–outbreak of Victoria flu is recorded among the patients and staff of a nursing home in Florida

4–Justice Department reveals that 104 damage claims have been filed against the Federal Government under PL 94–380; total value is almost $11 million

4–Califano announces that a special meeting will be held on Monday the 7th to discuss the moratorium and recommend a course of action for the remainder of the 1976–1977 flu season

4–Califano sends a memo to President Carter, summarizing the history of the moratorium, identifying the problem posed by the recent outbreak of Victoria flu, and stating his intention to meet with an *ad hoc* committee on Monday to discuss the options, after which he (Califano) would consult with the White House and make a decision; Califano closes by suggesting that he does not think the President should publicly make the decision

4–Representatives Henry Waxman and Andrew Maguire of Rogers' subcommittee hold a morning press conference at which they voice their concern over the administration and implementation of the program

4–HEW Undersecretary Hale Champion informs Sencer he will be replaced as head of CDC

7–Califano convenes an open meeting to discuss resumption of influenza vaccination; *ad hoc* panel of academic, scientific, political and media experts, chaired by John Knowles, meets at HEW; panel recommends that Califano resume vaccination of the high-risk group with bivalent vaccine, but reaches no agreement on general resumption

7–During meeting it becomes known that Califano wants Sencer's resignation as director of CDC; Sencer confirms

7–Acting General Counsel Barrett sends memo to Califano, enclosing the revised Informed Consent forms and advising that the Secretary invite comments thereon from Justice and from the National Commission for the Protection of Human Subjects

8–at a news conference, Califano announces that he is lifting the ban on bivalent and B Hong Kong vaccines to help combat small outbreaks of Victoria and Hong Kong flu; moratorium is continued on swine monovalent vaccine; mass outreach campaign is not to be resumed

9–health officials from a majority of states announce that bivalent vaccine will be made available to physicians and health clinics but that mass immunization programs will not be resumed

9–an AFEB Ad Hoc Subcommittee on Influenza submits recommendations on vaccination of armed forces for the spring; advises that recruits be given the swine-Victoria bivalent vaccine, but that as soon as Victoria monovalent vaccine should become available, recruits be given that only; AFEB accepts the recommendation

14–15–meeting is held at CDC with representatives of NIAID, BoB, and the Department of Agriculture to discuss swine flu in man and pigs and methods of control

MARCH 1977

11–Califano convenes an *ad hoc*, advisory panel to make suggestions and recommendations on flu vaccine policy for the next year; at end of all-day meeting, the group concludes that only high-risk group or those with important occupations (70 million in all) should be targets for flu vaccination next winter; vaccine will immunize against Victoria flu; swine flu vaccine is not recommended

D

SELECTED

DOCUMENTS

1. Sencer "action-memorandum," written March 13, 1976, dated March 18, from James F. Dickson for Theodore Cooper to HEW Secretary David Mathews.
2. Memorandum for OMB Director James T. Lynn, written and dated March 15, 1976, from HEW Secretary Mathews.
3. Memorandum for President Ford, undated, with talking points for March 22, 1976, meeting, from Budget Director Lynn, with two attachments:
   - Attachment A. "Uncertainties Surrounding a Federal Mass Swine Influenza Immunization Program."
   - Attachment B. The Sencer "action-memorandum" (as above).
4. CDC staff study on vaccine stockpiling, prepared in May, 1976, for use at subsequent advisory meetings.
5. Two-page consent form for the swine flu program, as actually used, with two second pages, one for monovalent and the other for bivalent vaccine.

MEMORANDUM

DEPARTMENT OF HEALTH, EDUCATION, AND WELFARE
OFFICE OF THE ASSISTANT SECRETARY FOR HEALTH

TO   : The Secretary
            Through: ES *MK* /*R* _____

DATE: MAR 18 1976

FROM   : Assistant Secretary for Health

SUBJECT: Swine Influenza--ACTION

ISSUE

How should the Federal Government respond to the influenza problem
caused by a new virus?

FACTS

1. In February 1976 a new strain of influenza virus, designated as
influenza A/New Jersey/76 (HswlN1), was isolated from an outbreak of
disease among recruits in training at Fort Dix, New Jersey.

2. The virus is antigenically related to the influenza virus which
has been implicated as the cause of the 1918-1919 pandemic which
killed 450,000 people--more than 400 of every 100,000 Americans.

3. The entire U.S. population under the age of 50 is probably
susceptible to this new strain.

4. Prior to 1930, this strain was the predominate cause of human
influenza in the U.S. Since 1930, the virus has been limited to
transmission among swine with only occasional transmission from swine
to man--with no secondary person-to-person transmission.

5. In an average year, influenza causes about 17,000 deaths (9 per
100,000 population) and costs the nation approximately $500 million.

6. Severe epidemics, or pandemics, of influenza occur at approximately
10 year intervals. In 1968-69, influenza struck 20 percent of our population,
causing more than 33,000 deaths (14 per 100,000) and cost an estimated
$3.2 billion.

7. A vaccine to protect against swine influenza can be developed before
the next flu season; however, the production of large quantities would
require extraordinary efforts by drug manufacturers.

The Secretary   2

ASSUMPTIONS

1. Although there has been only one outbreak of A/swine influenza,
person-to-person spread has been proven and additional outbreaks
cannot be ruled out. Present evidence and past experience indicate
a strong possibility that this country will experience widespread
A/swine influenza in 1976-77. Swine flu represents a major antigenic
shift from recent viruses and the population under 50 is almost universally
susceptible. These are the ingredients for a pandemic.

2. Routine public health influenza recommendations (immunization of the
population at high risk--elderly and chronically ill persons) would
not forestall a flu pandemic. Routine actions would have to be
supplemented.

3. The situation is one of "go or no go". If extraordinary measures
are to be undertaken there is barely enough time to assure adequate
vaccine production and to mobilize the nation's health care delivery
system. Any extensive immunization program would have to be in full
scale operation by the beginning of September and should not last beyond
the end of November 1976. A decision must be made now.

4. There is no medical epidemiologic basis for excluding any part of the
population--swine flu vaccine will be recommended for the total population
except in individual cases. Similarly there is no public health or
epidemiologic rationale for narrowing down the targeted population.
Further, it is assumed that it would be socially and politically unacceptable
to plan for less than 100 percent coverage. Therefore, it is assumed that
any recommendations for action must be directed toward the goal of
immunizing 213 million people in three months (September through November
1976). The nation has never attempted an immunization program of such
scope and intensity.

5. A public health undertaking of this magnitude cannot succeed without
Federal leadership, sponsorship, and some level of financial support.

6. The vaccine when purchased in large quantities will cost around
50 cents per dose. Nationally, the vaccine will cost in excess of
$100 million. To this total must be added delivery costs, as well as
costs related to surveillance and monitoring. Part, but not all, of the
costs can be considered sunk costs, or as non-additive. Regardless of
what strategy is adopted, it will be extremely difficult to estimate
the amount of additional costs that will result from a crash influenza
immunization program.

7. The Advisory Committee on Immunization Practices will recommend
formally and publicly, the immunization of the total U.S. population
against A/swine influenza.

8. Any recommended course of action, other than no action, must assure:

--that a supply of vaccine is produced which is adequate to immunize
the whole population.

--that adequate supplies of vaccine are available as needed at health
care delivery points.

--that the American people are made aware of the need for immunization
against this flu virus.

--that the population systematically reach or be reached by the
health system.

--that the Public Health Service maintain epidemiologic, laboratory,
and immunization surveillance of the population for complications
of vaccination, for influenza morbidity and mortality, and for
vaccine effectiveness and efficacy.

--that the unique research opportunities be maximized.

--that evaluation of the effectiveness of the efforts is conducted.

ALTERNATIVE COURSES OF ACTION

1. No Action

An argument can be made for taking no extraordinary action beyond what
would normally be recommended. To date there has been only one outbreak.
The swine flu virus has been around, but has not caused a problem among
humans since 1930.

Pro:

--The market place would prevail--private industry (drug manufacturers)
would produce in accordance with its estimate of demand and the
consumers would make their own decisions. Similarly, States would
respond in accordance with their own sets of priorities.

--The "pandemic" might not occur and the Department would have
avoided unnecessary health expenditures.

--Any real action would require direct Federal intervention which is
contrary to current administration philosophy.

The Secretary   4

Con:

--Congress, the media, and the American people will expect some action.

--The Administration can tolerate unnecessary health expenditures better than unnecessary death and illness, particularly if a flu pandemic should occur.

--In all likelihood, Congress will act on its own initiative.

2. Minimum Response

Under this option there would be a limited Federal role with primary reliance on delivery systems now in place and on spontaneous, non-governmental action.

a. The Federal Government would advise the drug industry to develop and produce A/swine vaccine sufficient to immunize the general population. The Federal Government would underwrite this effort by promising to purchase vaccine for the 58 million Federal beneficiaries.

b. A nationwide public awareness program would be undertaken to serve as general backdrop for local programs.

c. The Public Health Service would stimulate community programs sponsored by local organizations (medical societies, associations, industries, etc.)

d. The Center for Disease Control would maintain epidemiologic and laboratory surveillance of the population.

e. The National Institutes of Health would conduct studies and investigations, particularly on new and improved vaccines.

Pro:

--The approach is characterized by high visability, minimum Federal intervention, and diffused liability and responsibility. It is a partnership with the private sector that relies on Federal stimulation of nongovernmental action.

--The burden on the Federal budget would be minimal. Assuming purchase of vaccines for 58 million beneficiaries, plus additional costs related to c., d., and e., above the total new obligational authority requirement would not exceed $40 million ($32 million for vaccine; plus 8 million for surveillance, monitoring, evaluation, and research).

--Success would depend upon widespread voluntary action--in terms of individual choice to seek immunization and in terms of voluntary community programs not unlike the polio programs of the past.

Con:

--There is little assurance that vaccine manufacturers will undertake the massive production effort that would be required to assure availability of vaccine for the entire nation.

--There would be no control over the distribution of vaccines to the extent that they are available; the poor, the near poor, and the aging usually get left out. Even under routine flu recommendations in which the elderly are a primary target, only about half the high risk population gets immunized against flu.

--Probably only about half the population would get immunized.

3. Government Program

This alternative is based on virtually total government responsibility for the nationwide immunization program.

a. The Federal Government would advise vaccine manufacturers to embark on full scale production of vaccine with the expectation of Federal purchase of up to 200 million doses.

b. The Public Health Service, through the CDC would purchase the vaccines for distribution to State Health Departments.

c. In each State the health department would organize and carry out an immunization program designed to reach 100 percent of the State's population. Vaccine would be available only through programs carried out under the aegis of the State health department (or the Federal Government for direct Federal beneficiaries).

d. Primary reliance would be placed on systematic, planned delivery of vaccine in such a way as to make maximum use of intensive, high volume immunization techniques and procedures--particularly the use of jet-injector guns.

e. In addition to a general nationwide awareness program, intensive promotion and outreach activities would be carried out at the local level. Maximum use would be made of temporary employment of unemployed workers, high school and college students, housewives, and retired people as outreach workers and for jobs requiring no special health skills.

The Secretary   6

    f.   The Center for Disease Control would maintain epidemiologic and
        laboratory surveillance of the population.

    g.   The National Institutes of Health would conduct studies and
        investigations, particularly on new and improved vaccines.

    h.   The program would be evaluated to assess the effectiveness of the
        effort in reducing influenza associated morbidity, hospitalization,
        and mortality in a pandemic period.

Pro:

--Under this alternative adequate availability of vaccine would be
  closest to certainty, and the vaccine would be distributed throughout
  the nation most equitably.

--There would be greater certainty of participation of all States
  as well as a predictably more uniform level of intensity across the
  nation.

--Accessibility to immunization services would not depend upon
  economic status.

--This approach would provide the framework for better planning -
  for example, the use of travelling immunization teams which could
  take the vaccine to the people; and greater use of the jet injector,
  and other mass immunization techniques.

--The Federal and State governments traditionally have been responsible
  for the control of communicable diseases; therefore, the strategy
  relies upon government action in an area of public health where the
  States are strong and where basic operating mechanisms exist.

Con:

--This alternative would be very costly and given the timing, the
  magnitude of the problem, and the status of State fiscal health,
  the costs would have to be borne by the Federal Government. The
  impact on the Federal budget would be an increase of $190 million
  in new obligational authority.

--The approach is inefficient to the extent that it fails to take
  advantage of the private sector health delivery system, placing
  too much reliance on public clinics and government action.

--While this approach would undoubtedly result in a higher percentage
of the population being immunized than would be the case with the
Minimum Response strategy (alternative 2), it is unlikely that the
public sector could achieve uniform high levels of protection.
Although socioeconomic barriers to immunization services would
be virtually eliminated, breakdowns would occur because the program
is beyond the scope of official agencies.

--A totally "public" program is contrary to the spirit and custom
of health care delivery in this country and should only be
considered if it is clearly the most effective approach.

4. Combined Approach

A program based on this strategy would take advantage of the strengths
and resources of both the public and private sectors. Successful
immunization of our population in three months' time can be accomplished
only in this manner in this country. In essence, the plan would rely on:
the Federal Government for its technical leadership and coordination,
and its purchase power; State health agencies for their experience in
conducting immunization programs and as logical distribution centers
for vaccine; and on the private sector for its medical and other resources
which must be mobilized.

a. The Federal Government would advise vaccine manufacturers to
embark on full scale production of enough vaccine to immunize
the American people. The Public Health Service would contract
for 200 million doses of vaccine which would be made available
at no cost through State health agencies.

b. State health agencies would develop plans to immunize the people
in their States through a combination of official and voluntary
action - travelling immunization teams, community programs,
private physician practices, as examples.

c. The strategy would be to tailor the approach to the situation or
opportunity--using mass immunization techniques where appropriate,
but also using delivery points already in place such as:
physicians' offices, health department clinics, community health
centers--any place with the competence to perform immunization
services.

d. Awareness campaigns would be carried out at the local level against
a broader, generalized nationwide effort. Use would be made of
unemployed workers, students, etc., for certain jobs.

e. The Center for Disease Control would maintain epidemiologic and
laboratory surveillance of the population.

The Secretary   8

    f.   The National Institutes of Health would conduct studies and
        investigations of vaccine effectiveness and efficacy.

    g.   The program would be evaluated to assess the effectiveness of the
        effort in reducing influenza associated morbidity, hospitalization,
        and mortality in a pandemic period.

Pro:

--Under this alternative adequate availability of vaccine would be
  closest to certainty, and the vaccine would be distributed throughout
  the nation most equitably.

--There would be greater certainty of participation of all States
  as well as a predictably more uniform level of intensity across
  the nation.

--Accessibility to immunization services would not depend upon
  socioeconomic factors.

--Making use of all delivery points better assures that the vaccine
  will get to more people.

--The approach provides the framework for planning and expands the
  scope of resources which can be applied.

--Undertaking the program in this manner provides a practical,
  contemporary example of government, industry, and private citizens
  cooperating to serve a common cause.

Con:

--This strategy would require substantial Federal expenditures. A
  supplemental request of approximately $134 million would be needed.

--Under this alternative there is the greatest possibility of some
  people being needlessly reimmunized.

<u>DISCUSSION</u>

Any of the courses of action would raise budgetary and authorization
questions and these will be discussed later. More important is the question
of what the Federal Government is willing to invest if some action is
deemed necessary to avert a possible influenza pandemic. We have not
undertaken a health program of this scope and intensity before in our
history. There are no precedents, nor mechanisms in place that are suited

The Secretary   9

to an endeavor of this magnitude. Given this situation, can we afford
the administrative and programmatic inflexibility that would result from
normal considerations about duplicative costs, third party reimbursements,
and Federal-State or public-private relationships and responsibilities?
The magnitude of the challenge suggests that the Department must either
be willing to take extraordinary steps or be willing to accept an approach
to the problem that cannot succeed.

It is recommended that the Department, through the Public Health Service
and the Center for Disease Control, undertake an influenza immunization
campaign as outlined in alternative 4, Combined Approach. This alternative
best satisfies all of the minimum program requirements outlined earlier
and more importantly, it is the most likely to succeed--more people would
be protected.

The question of legislative authorization is not entirely clear. It
would appear that Section 311 a. of the Public Health Service Act contains
adequate authority to implement the recommended program. If 311 a. cannot
be used, then it will be necessary to seek "point of order" authority
in the supplemental appropriation act. It is anticipated that Congress
would be receptive to "point of order" language in this instance.

It will be necessary to seek a supplemental appropriation so that all
parties can begin to mobilize for the big push in the fall. It will also
be necessary for the funds to be available until expended because the
program, although time-limited, falls into fiscal year 1976, the transition
quarter, and fiscal year 1977. In general terms the request would be for
approximately $134 million made up as follows:

        Immunization Programs
           (vaccines, supplies, temporary personnel,
              awareness) $126 million

        Surveillance and Research   8 million

RECOMMENDATION

It is recommended that the Secretary adopt alternative 4 as the Department's
strategy and that the Public Health Service be given responsibility for
the program and be directed to begin immediate implementation.

                              Theodore Cooper, M.D.

March 15, 1976

MEMORANDUM FOR THE HONORABLE JAMES T. LYNN

There is evidence there will be a major flu epidemic this coming
fall. The indication is that we will see a return of the 1918 flu
virus that is the most virulent form of flu. In 1918 a half million
people died. The projections are that this virus will kill one
million Americans in 1976.

To have adequate protection, industry would have to be advised
now in order to have time to prepare the some 200 million doses
of vaccine required for mass inoculation. The decision will have
to be made in the next week or so. We will have a recommendation on this matter since a supplementary appropriation will be
required.

Today our two leading epidemiologists are here and are holding
a briefing after lunch on this subject. It might be most useful
for an appropriate member of your staff to attend. The briefing
will be at 2 p.m. in Room 5613 of the HEW North Building.

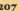

Secretary

EXECUTIVE OFFICE OF THE PRESIDENT
OFFICE OF MANAGEMENT AND BUDGET
WASHINGTON, D.C. 20503

SWINE INFLUENZA PROGRAM MEETING
Monday, March 22, 1976
11:00 to 11:30 a.m. (30 minutes)
Cabinet Room

From: James T. Lynn

I.   PURPOSE

To discuss a possible Federal initiative to immunize all
Americans against swine influenza.

II.   BACKGROUND PARTICIPANTS AND PRESS PLAN

A.   Background: HEW is concerned about a possible "outbreak" of swine influenza during the winter of 1976-
1977 and recommends a $134 million Federal program to
immunize every American. If this is to be done,
drug companies must be given the go-ahead to produce
the necessary vaccine within the next two weeks. The
decision to give the go-ahead to vaccine manufacturers
and to seek a 1976 budget supplemental is complicated
by both uncertainties and its precedential implications.

-- Attachment A outlines some of the uncertainties
within which this decision must be made.

-- Attachment B is an HEW memorandum on the subject.

B.   Participants: Secretary Mathews; HEW Assistant Secretar
Ted Cooper and his deputy, Jim Dickson; Richard Cheney,
James Lynn, James Cannon and Paul O'Neill.

C.   Press Plan: None

III.   TALKING POINTS

A.   Mr. Secretary, would you please start off by explaining:

1.   What swine influenza is and how it can be distinguished from other types of flu in terms of
its severity?

2.   What is the probability of an occurrence of an
epidemic in the winter of 1976-1977, given the
10-year cycle of epidemics, the last of which
occurred in the 1968/1969 winter?

3.   Why do we believe that the very same swine influenza
virus that was recently identified in New Jersey
will cause a nationwide epidemic this coming
winter as opposed to say, a mutant form of this
virus or another virus?

Attachment A

Uncertainties Surrounding a Federal
Mass Swine Influenza Immunization Program

-- <u>Scientifice Evidence on Likelihood and Success of Immunization</u>:
Person-to-person transmission of the swine virus has been
proven in only one location, Fort Dix in New Jersey. Further
scientific evidence on the probability of an occurrence of
swine flu virus next year may or may not become available
before the current flu season is over. HEW epidemiologists
have stated that the probability is "unknown."

The swine virus is a different strain entirely from the
flus of the past few years. The swine flu vaccine will
have no effect whatever on preventing these more conventional flus. Moreover, there remains a possibility that
mutated swine virus may occur -- against which the vaccine
to be developed would not be effective.

-- <u>Seriousness of Swine Influenza</u>: The number of Americans
that would be seriously ill or killed if an epidemic did
occur may not be analogous to the 1919 experience of 500,000
deaths because of the absence in 1919 of antibiotics. We
cannot be certain that there have been no person-to-person
transmission of swine influenza since 1930.

-- <u>Implications of a Federal Initiative</u>: Will it be necessary
to mount another massive Federal effort in each succeeding
year (1) if the swine influenza epidemic does not occur in
the winter of 1976/1977 or (2) in order to protect every
American against mutating versions of swine virus?

-- <u>Press Attention</u>: The national press is already aware of
a possible swine influenza occurence through weekly HEW
press conferences on the flu morbidity.

-- <u>Views of the Scientific Community</u>: HEW is now in the
process of trying to obtain consensus from all important
members of the virology scientific community on the advis-
ability of a nationwide immunization drive against the
swine flu virus. Nevertheless, what is the contrary virology
argument against the massive immunizations?

COPY

ANALYSIS OF VACCINE STOCKPILE OPTION CENTER FOR DISEASE CONTROL*

One of the options discussed at the CDC very early after the Fort Dix outbreak was to produce the monovalent A/New Jersey vaccine and stockpile until further evidence of virus spread. This option was again considered at the ACIP meetings on March 10 and May 6. The consensus on all three of these occasions was that stockpiling is not an acceptable alternative to a complete and fully committed vaccination program. In more recent weeks the issue of stockpiling has re-emerged. Reevaluation of this option is the subject of this report. To facilitate analysis we have made the following four basic assumptions:

(1) Bivalent vaccine (including some monovalent) would be distributed in 1976 for "high risk" groups as planned, presumably in the early fall.
(2) Monovalent A/New Jersey vaccine would be stockpiled at the state or local level.
(3) Materials would be accumulated and well-trained key personnel would be placed on a standby basis at the national, state, and local level.
(4) Evidence of reappearance of swine influenza-like virus in humans would trigger the remobilization of resources and begin the nationwide immunization program.

The concept of stockpiling has been considered on the basis of feasibility and costs in terms of dollars and time for each of the following three major elements of the program:

A. VACCINE STORAGE

Present FDA regulations list the expiration date of vaccines as 18 months after the date of bottling. This regulation is designed largely to prevent the use of outdated vaccine in the event of an antigenic drift or shift. Considerable evidence suggests that the vaccine may be stored under proper conditions at $4^{\circ}C$ without loss of potency for 3 years, and probably longer.

1. Dollar cost

A mixture of 10- and 50-dose vials packaged and ready for distribution requires 1 cu. ft. for 5,000 doses, or 32,000 cu. ft. of storage for 160 million doses.

---

*As submitted to House of Representatives, Committee on Interstate and Foriegn Commerce, Subcommittee on Health and the Environment, 94th Congress, Second Session, June 28, 1976 Supplemental Hearings, Serial No. 94-113, p. 9-11.

The cost in Atlanta for maximum security storage under con-
trolled refrigeration is 60¢ per cu. ft. per month. Assuming this
to be an average price throughout the country, storage costs for
the vaccine would be $20,000 per month or approximately $240,000
per year.

2. Time cost

The vaccine could be delivered to the state or local
grantees as per present contract with manufacturers, resulting
in 62 storage points. An alternative would be for the Federal
Government to maintain control and storage of the vaccine at
selected sites throughout the country. Distribution from these
sites may require more time, however. Distribution of the vaccine from the 62 or more storage points to designated vaccination
sites and private physicians would require a minimum of 1 to 2
weeks.

B. STANDBY PROGRAM ORGANIZATION

Before placing the immunization program on a standby basis,
all organizational plans and training sessions will have been
completed and all project grantees will have had experience in
conducting the bivalent vaccine campaign. Temporary employees
would be released and other state or local public health employees detailed to the vaccine program would return to regular
jobs. To restart the program would require a well-trained "disaster relief" team consisting of key permanent personnel capable
of quickly training newly-hired or assigned personnel to perform
essential program functions such as clerical duties, operation of
the jet gun, and gun repair.

1. Dollar cost

Much of the present $26 million allocation to grantees
would be spent on present organization, training, and delivery
of bivalent vaccine. Additional monies would be requested for
training new personnel, which may consist of as much as 50% of
the total program staff. Additional personnel and training costs
may approach $6 million. The cost for a second publicity cam-
paign at the time of the decision to "go" is unknown. Free
publicity from the report of new virus outbreaks may lessen the
need for publicly supported publicity campaigns.

2. Time cost

Initiating the "disaster plan" publicity, and the hiring
and training of new personnel for the vaccination program is
estimated to require a minimum of 2 to 4 weeks.

C.   PROGRAM RESPONSIVENESS

As presently planned, most of the vaccine would be administered by jet injector. Additional jet injector guns would be needed since the number of vaccinations given per day would increase under the stockpile option. These guns can be manufactured and delivered.

1.   Dollar cost

The major direct cost would be $1 million for 1,000 more guns. At present, 3,000 guns are to be available on September 1.

2.   Time cost

To vaccinate 160 million people with 4,000 guns would require 40 days, or approximately seven 6-day weeks. This does not, of course, account for vaccine given by needle and syringe, which may require a longer period to complete.

D.   CONCLUSION

Obstacles to the stockpiling concept and "disaster relief plan" are not insurmountable. The vaccine could be stored and a qualified team which is capable of responding quickly to an epidemic threat could be maintained if the federal, state and local public health authorities were committed to the program. However, with time, very likely that commitment would become less, key personnel would be lost through reorganization and attrition, and program effectiveness would decrease.

The total cost of stockpiling the vaccine and delaying the program for 1 year would be approximately $7-8 million. Not included in this figure would be the cost of an "all-out" virus surveillance program. Part of this cost would be diverted from the present $26 million allocation to project grantees, but many of the 62 grantees are unlikely to agree to the concept of stockpiling without an established mechanism for providing additional funds to cover at least a portion of the above cost. If we can assume for purposes of this report that the Administration and the Congress would agree to additional appropriations, cost also ceases to be an obstacle. The whole issue of stockpiling then becomes a question of time. Can we afford to wait for additional evidence of virus spread before beginning the campaign?

Only 2 years in modern times, 1957 and 1968, can serve as models for predicting the spread of pandemic influenza in the continental U.S.A. The period from the first virus isolation to the first outbreak in the civilian population was 3 weeks in 1957 and 7 weeks in 1968; from virus isolation to documented outbreak in one-third or more of the States was 10 weeks in 1957 and 12 weeks in 1968; from isolation to peak activity was 14 weeks in 1957 and 15 weeks in 1968.

Assuming that an additional 2 weeks are required to produce a protective antibody response after vaccination, the vaccine must be given 1 to 5 weeks after the first virus isolation in order to prevent the first outbreak. This is clearly not possible. The longer the time after 1 to 5 weeks which is required to administer the vaccine, the less effective the program will be. However, if we consider a more modest goal, such as interruption of the pandemic before outbreaks occur in one-third of the States, more time is available. But even to achieve this, vaccination must be completed 8 to 10 weeks after first evidence of virus isolation. According to our estimates above, to complete the vaccination program from the signal "go" would require a minimum of 9-11 weeks. A few smaller, highly urbanized States may require less time. Many may require more. Thus, some States could probably achieve this goal. But in our view, a goal which accepts success in only less populated States cannot be adopted as national policy.

In this report we have consciously attempted to avoid bias by using minimal estimates of dollar and time costs. We have not, for example, considered the additional time which may be required to confirm the next swine influenza-like virus isolation or outbreak, the diminished impact of the initial $135 million investment of public funds, or the morbidity and mortality from early sporadic outbreaks. On the other hand, by our use of 1957 and 1968 as models we may have overestimated the speed at which the virus might spread. We have no real basis for predicting the epidemic behavior of the swine-like virus. Never before has an antigenic shift been detected so early or associated with such a limited outbreak. Quite likely, the longer the time before the next swine virus isolation, the longer the period of warning before a major epidemic. But we cannot be sure. Therefore, at present there is no acceptable alternative to a complete and fully committed vaccination program.

Important Information from the U.S. Public Health Service about Swine Flu and Victoria Flu Vaccines

INTRODUCTION

You probably have heard a good deal about swine flu and swine flu vaccine. You may know, for example, that swine flu caused an outbreak of several hundred cases at Ft. Dix, New Jersey, early in 1976– and that before then swine flu had not caused outbreaks among people since the 1920's.

With the vast majority of Americans being susceptible to swine flu, it is possible that there could be an epidemic this winter. No one can say for sure. However, if an epidemic were to break out, millions of people could get sick. Therefore, a special swine flu vaccine has been prepared and tested which should protect most people who receive it.

Certain people, such as those with chronic medical problems and the elderly, need annual protection against flu. Therefore, besides protection against swine flu, they also need protection against another type of flu (Victoria flu) that was around last winter and could occur again this winter. A separate vaccine has been prepared to give them protection against both types of flu.

These vaccines have been field tested and shown to produce very few side effects. Some people who receive the vaccine had fever and soreness during the first day or two after vaccination. These tests and past experience with other flu vaccines indicate that anything more severe than this would be highly unlikely.

Many people ask questions about flu vaccination during pregnancy. An advisory committee of the Public Health Service examined this question and reported that "there are no data specifically to contraindicate vaccination with the available killed virus vaccine in pregnancy. Women who are pregnant should be considered as having essentially the same balance of benefits and risks regarding influenza vaccination and influenza as the general population."

As indicated, some individuals will develop fever and soreness after vaccination. If you have more severe symptoms or if you have fever which lasts longer than a couple of days after vaccination, please consult your doctor or a health worker wherever you receive medical care.

While there is no reason to expect more serious reactions to this flu vaccination, persons who believe that they have been injured by this vaccination may have a claim. The Congress recently passed a law providing that such claims, with certain exceptions, may be filed only against the United States Government. Information regarding the filing of claims may be obtained by writing to the U.S. Public Health Service Claims Office, Parklawn Building, 5600 Fishers Lane, Rockville, Maryland 20852.

Attached is more information about flu and flu vaccine. Please take the time to read it carefully. You will be asked to sign a form indicating that you understand this information and that you consent to vaccination.

IMPORTANT INFORMATION
ABOUT SWINE INFLUENZA (FLU) VACCINE
(MONOVALENT)

July 15, 1976

The Disease

Influenza (flu) is caused by viruses. When people get flu they may have fever, chills, headache, dry cough or muscle aches. Illness may last several days or a week or more, and complete recovery is usual. However, complications may lead to pneumonia or death in some people. For the elderly and people with diabetes or heart, lung, or kidney diseases, flu may be especially serious.

It is unlikely that you have adequate natural protection against swine flu, since it has not caused widespread human outbreaks in 45 years.

The Vaccine

The vaccine will not give you flu because it is made from killed viruses. Today's flu vaccines cause fewer side effects than those used in the past. In contrast with some other vaccines, flu vaccine can be taken safely during pregnancy.

One shot will protect most people from swine flu during the next flu season; however, either a second shot or a different dosage may be required for persons under age 25. If you are under 25 and a notice regarding such information is not attached, this information will be provided to you wherever you receive the vaccine.

Possible Vaccine Side Effects

Most people will have no side effects from the vaccine. However, tenderness at the site of the shot may occur and last for several days. Some people will also have fever, chills, headache, or muscle aches within the first 48 hours.

Special Precautions

As with any vaccine or drug, the possibility of severe or potentially fatal reactions exists. However, flu vaccine has rarely been associated with severe or fatal reactions. In some instances people receiving vaccine have had allergic reactions. You should note very carefully the following precautions:

- Children under a certain age should not routinely receive flu vaccine. Please ask about age limitations if this information is not attached.
- People with known allergy to eggs should receive the vaccine only under special medical supervision.
- People with fever should delay getting vaccinated until the fever is gone.
- People who have received another type of vaccine in the past 14 days should consult a physician before taking the flu vaccine.

If you have any questions about flu or flu vaccine, please ask.

REGISTRATION FORM

I have read the above statement about swine flu, the vaccine, and the special precautions. I have had an opportunity to ask questions, including questions regarding vaccination recommendations for persons under age 25, and understand the benefits and risks of flu vaccination. I request that it be given to me or to the person named below of whom I am the parent or guardian.

INFORMATION ON PERSON TO RECEIVE VACCINE		FOR CLINIC USE
Name (Please Print)	Birthdate Age	
Address	County of Residence	Clinic Ident.
		Date Vaccinated
		Manufacturer and Lot No.

Signature of person to receive vaccine or Parent or Guardian   Date

CDC 7.31
7-76

U.S. Department of Health, Education, and Welfare / Public Health Service / Center for Disease Control / Atlanta, Georgia 30333

IMPORTANT INFORMATION ABOUT
SWINE AND VICTORIA INFLUENZA (FLU) VACCINE
(BIVALENT)

July 15, 1976

The Disease
Influenza (flu) is caused by viruses. When people get flu they may have fever, chills, headache, dry cough or muscle aches. Illness may last several days or a week or more, and complete recovery is usual. However, complications may lead to pneumonia or death in some people. For the elderly and people with diabetes or heart, lung, or kidney diseases, flu may be especially serious.

It is unlikely that you have adequate protection against swine flu, since it has not caused widespread human outbreaks in the past 45 years. You may or may not have adequate protection against Victoria flu, although many Americans had this flu last winter. It was responsible for over 12,000 deaths.

The Vaccine
The vaccine will not give you flu because it is made from killed viruses. Today's flu vaccines cause fewer side effects than those used in the past. In contrast with some other vaccines, flu vaccine can be taken safely during pregnancy.

One shot will protect most people from swine and Victoria flu during the next flu season; however, either a second shot or a different dosage may be required for persons under age 25. If you are under 25 and a notice regarding such information is not attached, this information will be provided to you wherever you receive the vaccine.

Possible Vaccine Side Effects
Most people will have no side effects from the vaccine. However, tenderness at the site of the shot may occur and last for several days. Some people will also have fever, chills, headache, or muscle aches within the first 48 hours.

Special Precautions
As with any vaccine or drug, the possibility of severe or potentially fatal reactions exists. However, flu vaccine has rarely been associated with severe or fatal reactions. In some instances people receiving vaccine have had allergic reactions. You should note very carefully the following precautions:

- Children under a certain age should not routinely receive flu vaccine. Please ask about age limitations if this information is not attached.
- People with known allergy to eggs should receive the vaccine only under special medical supervision.
- People with fever should delay getting vaccinated until the fever is gone.
- People who have received another type of vaccine in the past 14 days should consult a physician before taking the flu vaccine.

If you have any questions about flu or flu vaccine, please ask.   ☆USGPO: 1976 — 216-225

REGISTRATION FORM

I have read the above statement about swine and Victoria flu, the vaccine, and the special precautions. I have had an opportunity to ask questions, including questions regarding vaccination recommendations for persons under age 25, and understand the benefits and risks of flu vaccination. I request that it be given to me or to the person named below of whom I am the parent or guardian.

INFORMATION ON PERSON TO RECEIVE VACCINE		FOR CLINIC USE
Name (Please Print)	Birthdate Age	Clinic Ident.
Address	County of Residence	Date Vaccinated
Signature of person to receive vaccine or Parent or Guardian Date		Manufacturer and Lot No.

CDC 7.32
7-76   U.S. Department of Health, Education, and Welfare / Public Health Service / Center for Disease Control / Atlanta, Georgia 30333

E

USEFUL

QUESTIONS

In this appendix we offer a set of questions we think useful in reviewing influenza prospects and programs. They are intended to elaborate the assumptions underlying initial decisions and to lay a base for program review. The questions deal with the magnitude of the potential influenza threat, the desirability, feasibility and scope of a responsive program, and its implementation. Detailed questions on implementation become increasingly important the larger the contemplated Federal role and the wider the program's scope.

We doubt that anyone would want to ask all questions of any single expert group, no matter what its expertise. We do think the last question should be asked of every group, regardless of expertise.

A. The threat of influenza in the United States

1. How likely is the new influenza strain to spread in the United States? What do you consider the likelihood of no outbreak, of sporadic outbreaks only, of an epidemic? Within what time?

2. What number of people (grouped according to age, medical condition or socioeconomic class) are likely to get influenza? What number are likely to die from it? On what assumptions? What protection already exists in the population? What protection, if any, would be retained from previous vaccination?

3. What additional surveillance, if any, should be undertaken to identify the appearance and magnitude of influenza outbreaks?

B. Vaccination and alternative interventions

1. Would you recommend any substitutes or supplements to vaccination with killed virus vaccine (e.g., live vaccine, amantadine, other agents)? In what circumstances would you advocate their use at present? Air assumptions.

2. Against what viral strains should the production of vaccine be contemplated? What do you consider the relative advantages and disadvantages of whole and split virus vaccines? Is there a role for both? Under what assumptions?

C. Availability and testing vaccine

1. What vaccines are already available? What is known about their possible usefulness?

2. Is manufacture of new vaccines feasible, and how long will it take to produce what quantities? What are your assumptions about facilities, final dosage and yield at each stage of production? Which steps limit the volume and rate of production? How readily changed, if at all, is each rate-limiting step? What are the tradeoffs (e.g., cost, reactivity)?

3. What quality control and other testing must be done at each stage of production?

4. What field trials should be conducted, with what dosages and types of vaccine, what number of doses, and in which population groups?

D. Vaccine benefits, risks and costs

1. What efficacy in terms of disease prevention and decreased mortality do you expect from the new vaccine, for which age groups? How long will it take for inoculation to confer protection, and how long-lasting will it be? Air assumptions.

2. What side effects, of what type and severity, and in what frequency, do you foresee?

3. What additional surveillance will be required to detect different types and frequencies of side effects?

4. What do you estimate as the dollar cost of vaccine production and administration? What are the components of your estimate? Are there additional, indirect costs, as from litigation, which you anticipate? Air your assumptions.

E. Program objectives, organization, implementation

1. What vaccination objectives would you recommend in terms of total numbers to be vaccinated, dosages and schedules in different age groups, reaching what socioeconomic levels, over what time span, completed by when? State what you would like ideally. Then state what you would regard as satisfactory. Air your assumptions.

2. Given these aims, what alternatives do you see for administration of the following tasks as among federal, state and local agencies, private manufacturers, insurers, medical practitioners, voluntary agencies, other (specify in each case)?
   - Preparing recombinant and seed strains
   - Producing and distributing vaccine
   - Purchase of vaccine
   - Testing vaccine at different stages
   - Storage of vaccine
   - Design and conduct of field trials
   - Surveillance of disease, vaccinations and side effects
   - Intergovernmental consultation (among whom?)
   - Advising doctors and professional societies

- Informing public interest groups and voluntary agencies (whom do you think relevant?)
- Assuming liability (for what?)
- Preparing consent forms
- Operational planning (e.g., ensuring local availability of consent forms, obtaining supplies, securing staff and space, giving injections)
- Explaining coincidences
- Statistical reporting
- Periodic program review

Do you foresee other tasks? Add them on.

3. Under each set of alternatives you give for handling these tasks, how many people do you expect will actually be inoculated? With what biases in terms of age, race, socioeconomic class and health risk? Air your assumptions.

4. What combinations of tasks and agencies do you recommend? Explain your reasons.

5. Who should be consulted in Congress? In what sequence? At what stages? By whom? Given the projected cost and program organization, what would be specifically required by way of legislative authorization and appropriations?

6. Working step-by-step backward from inoculation, what is required of each implementing agency? What are the weak links? Is there a hint of any issue just beneath the surface which could rise to haunt, slow or stop your preferred program (as liability did in 1976)?

7. How should HEW be organized internally to play its part? How linked to Department of Defense? Domestic Policy Staff? Veterans Administration? World Health Organization? Who has to do what, specifically? How minimize Congressional or press confusion about "who's in charge here," as occurred at times in 1976?

8. With what other top managements, public *or* private, should HEW prepare to deal directly, so as to avoid surprises like insurance company decision-making in 1976? Specifically, who should deal with whom, where and how?

9. What is expected of, by, from the media? On what premises? What steps should be taken to anticipate and relate technical contingencies, such as temporally linked deaths, to prospective media coverage?

10. How do you think the program you prefer should be presented to Congress, states, the medical community and media? As "available," "desirable" or "imperative"? For whom? Air assumptions.

F. Preparation for program review

1. List perceived deadlines for decision and action. When must what be done? Why? Which deadlines may be movable? Which not? Air assumptions.
2. When and how should the above questions and answers be reviewed? What should be the mechanism for review, given perceived deadlines and the development of additional information, whether anticipated or unexpected?
3. What new information would cause you to change some or all of the recommendations you have made? Which recommendations? In what ways changed? Air your assumptions.

PART TWO

NEW

DEVELOPMENTS

AND

TEACHING

14

LATER

DEVELOPMENTS

In Chapter 11, Legacies, and in Chapter 13, the Technical Afterword, we summarized developments in Federal immunization policy, legislation, scientific knowledge and the disease itself from the end of the swine flu program in 1977 to submission of our report in 1978. Four more years have passed. We now report on what has happened in the interval.

Immunization Policy

In 1978 CDC, with Califano's backing, sought to add to Federal immunization initiatives a permanent flu program. This was finally funded for a first year in September 1978, at half the preferred size. Just over $8 million instead of $15 million (the OMB-approved request) was included by the Senate and accepted by the House in a supplemental appropriation bill which President Carter signed September 8. Most of the money went to the states in grants for vaccination programs that winter.

But congressional action had been reluctant. The appropriation was killed once on the House floor, and its authorization was resisted stoutly in the Senate by the ranking Republican on the Health Subcommittee, Senator Richard Schweiker of Pennsylvania. In both Houses the complaint was the same. As Schweiker put it to the Senate, August 4, 1978:

It really is sort of ironic. We just came through the worst medical disaster in history in terms of modern technology, and you want to give them a prize for what has been done. . . .[81]

Opposition was renewed in 1979, although another $8 million eventually was squeezed out for a second year, and opponents prevailed in 1980 when no further funds were granted. The Federal influenza immunization initiative came to at least a temporary halt that year. And at the year's end the incoming President, Ronald Reagan, named Schweiker Secretary of Health and Human Services (HHS having succeeded HEW). "Temporary" promises to last a long time.

In 1981, far from restoring funds for flu, the Reagan Administration cut by 25 percent the grants for more traditional immunization initiatives, measles and the like. The states were cutting back as well. This left influenza at the top of no one's list, although Califano himself continues to argue for a long-term program in his recent memoir, *Governing America*.[82]

In our report to Califano we wrote that even without congressional endorsement, flu would still be part of more agendas than before. Obviously, this did not ensure continued movement toward a lasting program. Influenza now seems lower on government priority lists than at any time in many years. To some extent this may reflect the credibility gap of 1976—although CDC has enjoyed some public successes since, isolating the organism that causes Legionnaire's Disease and tracing risks of toxic shock syndrome to use of tampons.[83] Credibility aside, the fate of Federal influenza immunization certainly reflects the current political climate: less Washington initiative, more state responsibility and greater reliance on private enterprise.

Liability and Litigation

Since our last report, nothing much has happened to the issue of liability legislation at the Federal level. California has passed its own law, but in Washington, D.C., the issue remains where we left it: unresolved at HHS, unsettled on Capitol Hill. Califano stalled it and the heat has since gone out of it, lacking the fuel of Federal vaccination schemes or fresh emergencies. The Donaldson report, shorn of recommendations, remains on file with the subcommittees concerned and somewhere in the General Counsel's office at HHS there probably exists the original draft, recommendations and all. The new Secretary was acquainted with the issue as a Senator; his intentions, if any, are unknown to us.

Early in 1980, the House Interstate and Foreign Commerce Committee asked the Congressional Office of Technology Assessment (OTA) to prepare a report on a federal compensation program for vaccine-related injuries. The OTA argues briefly that some form of federal compensation program is desirable and discusses five elements the Congress would need to consider in any legislation: the vaccines included, the injuries covered, the extent and form of compensation, administrative mechanisms, and relations to other remedies, such as lawsuits. The OTA released its technical memorandum in November 1980.[84] Clearly written and comprehensive, no doubt it too is appropriately filed.

Meanwhile, in the Claims Division of the Justice Department, a group of twelve attorneys proceeds year by year to process claims and to defend the government in court against suits brought under the law of 1976. The pace has been slow, deliberately so; Justice sees its task as to protect the Treasury, not to ease the path for plaintiffs. Of nearly 1,500 suits thus far, two-thirds are still pending, although all but 111 of 4000 claims have been resolved. While total damages alleged in suits amounted to $2 billion and in claims to almost $3 billion, only $20 million had been actually awarded and paid out by May 1981.

While still in office, Califano was aggrieved by the slow pace and tried to speed it. He has argued since that the Justice Department attorneys were "dragging their feet. . . ."[85] Perhaps so. We know nothing to suggest that under Reagan they will alter their approach. Savings on awards will be offset in part by the administrative costs for those twelve lawyers.

Influenza Virus and Disease

Two recent scientific achievements dramatically extend our understanding of the influenza virus's genetic composition and antigenic structure. Using recombinant-DNA techniques, scientists have analyzed the complete chemical sequence of the RNA genes that produce hemagglutinin and neuraminidase.[86] This is a necessary step toward discovering the precise genetic determinants of infectivity and virulence in the virus. At the same time, other researchers have successfully crystallized the hemagglutinin protein, depicted its three-dimensional structure, and identified likely antigenic sites.[87] This breakthrough can lead to more specific understanding of the interactions between antibodies and the hemagglutinin antigens, and between the hemagglutinin molecule and surface receptors for the influenza virus. Additional research has elucidated the specific genetic determinants of several flu-virus components and has defined more precisely than before the antigenic relations among various types of influenza viruses.[88]

While molecular understanding of the influenza virus has become more solid in the past three years, the clinical and epidemiological behavior of the virus remains as slippery as ever.

In previous years, illness from the B influenza virus tended to be sporadic and relatively mild; in these respects the 1979–1980 flu season was startling. That year, a variant B virus (B/Singapore/79) caused surprisingly severe outbreaks of influenza in many parts of the United States. In fact, during that same flu season, the B virus was the predominant strain of influenza in this country.[89] New evidence abounds on the potential virulence of B virus in previously healthy victims.[90] Clinically, it did everything the A virus does.

In the spring of 1980, a variant of Victoria flu, the type A virus strain (H3N2) that had been dominant through most of the 1970's, once again became the most prevalent cause of influenza under the name Bangkok. But the Russian strain of A virus (H1N1) that had disappeared in the mid-1950's and re-emerged in 1977 continued to cause substantial amounts of illness in young adults. Both these viruses have drifted, year by year, but neither has been able to dominate the other in the human populations under attack. The duality defies our previous understanding of how A virus behaved. During the four flu seasons since 1978–1979, recommended vaccine for the general public in this country has been trivalent, containing antigens representative of both H3N2 and H1N1, along with the B virus.

While the two A viruses vied for dominance in the United States and elsewhere, a third type (H2N2) reportedly was isolated in the spring of 1980 in an outbreak among Soviet children in Leningrad.[91] It has been found nowhere else and soon disappeared there. Apparently as at Fort Dix, an antigenic shift occurred and rapidly disappeared, unable to dominate or even coexist with other strains in the vicinity.

Thus influenza continues to confound those who study it. The past three years have taught new respect for the B virus, raised questions about the frequency of sporadic appearances by different types of A virus, and witnessed widespread, simultaneous existence of two distinct A strains in the population. These findings underscore again how much we have to learn about the flu.

Prevention and Control

Immunization with killed-virus vaccine remains the mainstay of influenza prevention in the United States, although its efficacy is still controversial. Research continues on live-virus vaccines, and the drug amantadine has gained more recognition as an adjunct to immunization for the prevention and early treatment of type A flu.[92] The antigenic potential of vaccines is now assayed by reliable immunologic methods rather than by the less direct CCA units.[93] The new methods measure the amount of hemagglutinin antigen in vaccines, but do not assure their clinical effectiveness.

Clinical studies question the ability of recent vaccines to prevent disease, especially in comparison with the immunity conferred by natural infection.[94] An antibody response following immunization may not be very protective against a virus that has drifted, and the A virus still manages to drift with disarming frequency: the H3N2 Port Chalmers drifted into Victoria in 1976, Victoria into Texas in 1977, Texas into Bangkok in 1979. But doubts about the efficacy of flu vaccine are nothing new and recent research leaves most experts still endorsing vaccination for high-risk groups.[95] A stronger dose might be more effective. The ACIP recommendations for 1981–1982 double the antigenic content of the 1980–1981 trivalent vaccine.[96]

Since discovering a statistically significant relation between swine flu vaccination and Guillain-Barré syndrome, CDC has tracked the occurrence of this disorder among persons who do and do not receive flu immunizations. During the 1978–1979 and 1979–1980 flu seasons, the risk of Guillain-Barré syndrome did not appear to be significantly higher among influenza vaccinees than among others.[97] The added risk in 1976, associated with the swine flu program, had not been restricted to vaccine from any one manufacturer and the specific cause for increased incidence of this rare malady in vaccinated persons that year still remains a mystery.[98]

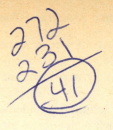

15

USES FOR

TEACHING

The original edition of this book has been used in different ways for a variety of teaching purposes. So has a separate teaching case done for our colleague Laurence Lynn from our report and records—and from reinterviews—as a one-day assignment in his course. Others use Lynn's text along with portions of our own. For that reason we include the bulk of it in this edition as Chapter 16.

It is because these materials serve the purposes of teachers and students that we proceeded to this new edition. We summarize below the classroom uses with which we have grown familiar from our own teaching and from exchanges with other instructors. Many adaptations are conceivable; we leave those to our readers who will understand their own curricular needs better than we can.

What follows is less than a "teaching note" in the full sense. Conventionally, a note that details the full plan for any given class, including the precise use of assignments, is published separately from the case itself. Students read the latter without reading the former. We think the convention a good one and we honor it. Here, we merely summarize key issues raised or questions posed by teachers to students. These are mostly students at professional schools in public health or medicine or journalism or public policy and management. Undergraduate uses are labeled as such.

We offer our summaries under six headings reflecting general purposes for which such courses are taught.

Quantitative Methods for Policy Analysis

The formal technique called decision analysis is a systematic, quantitative approach to weighing decisions. It is widely taught now in graduate programs of public policy, administration, business, medicine and public health. It is a valuable discipline, and the swine flu case offers a real-world situation that can illustrate both its strengths and its limitations.

Swine flu problems are grist for the decision-analytic mill. Three elements in any situation spark the interest of decision analysts: uncertainty, unavoidable decisions, and tradeoffs among valued outcomes. Uncertainty permeates the 1976 affair: How likely is an epidemic? How severe? How effective is the vaccine? How many people will be immunized? What are the risks of inoculation? And so forth. Some decisions cannot be avoided: even choosing to do nothing except wait and watch would have been as decisive as launching a national effort. And every choice runs headlong into tradeoffs: for one, the health of vaccinees exposed to unknown side effects versus their health unvaccinated in an epidemic; or for another, economic benefits and costs; or for a third, the pros and cons of credibility.

Every decision analysis is grounded in values. From the outset the analyst asks—and therefore the teacher does likewise—"Who is the decision-maker?" From whose vantage point are the pros and cons to be measured? Differently placed decision-makers very often see the problem somewhat differently and weigh the consequences on a different scale. In a famous phrase, "Where you stand depends on where you sit." Students are expected to take notice.

The swine flu situation illustrates a wide range of perspectives, all of which are relevant from some standpoint or other in a complicated, social-policy problem. One viewpoint espoused by some decision-makers is that of society as a whole. In deciding a national immunization program, what, on balance, is best for the country? What are the risks in the short run and in the long run? How can the economic or resource costs be measured against the expected benefits? How judge administrative feasibility? What, in sum, is the cost-effectiveness of the proposed program? At an opposite extreme there is the viewpoint of the individuals deciding whether or not to get flu shots. Students are asked to think about the differences between the negative value an individual would place on ten days of flu compared to the social cost of that same illness. How do the economic effects of immunization look to an individual as compared to society?

In between society and the individual are a host of other decision-makers: scientists, public officials, physicians, not to mention vaccine manufacturers and insurers. How do their perceptions and values differ from one another? On balance, which among the decision-makers best represents the abstract interests of society? The President? Legislators? Public health officials? Consumer representatives? Academic analysts? For that matter, are practicing physicians advising about shots still better agents for their patients? If so, why? One teacher finds it an instructive exercise for students to describe the 1976 situation from several different perspectives, tracing similarities and differences in the features included, and noting the importance attached to each.[99] Does decision analysis determine which perspective is the "right" one or, in practical terms, whose interests will prevail? Obviously not.

A logical next question becomes whether, at what points, and how a formal, quantitative analysis might have been helpful in 1976. What sort of analysis should have been done, prepared by whom, presented to whom? Would a formal analysis have pointed to a contingent strategy: make the vaccine and be prepared, but do no more until more is known? With the underpinning of analysis might such a strategy have had any more appeal than "stockpiling"? And was there time for more analysis had it been sought by Sencer? By Cooper? Morrill? Mathews? Cavanaugh? Lynn? Ford?

A notable feature of decision-making throughout the swine flu program is the absence of expressed, quantitative estimates about the probability of a pandemic. To a decision analyst, *subjective* probabilities are entirely appropriate. To most of the scientists and officials involved in the swine flu program, they were anathema. Probabilities rooted in empirical evidence are readily defended; not so those based upon subjective judgment. Should scientists prepare to volunteer subjective probabilities? Or resist like Cooper? Should Sencer have insisted on explicit probabilities from his staff and advisers? Should Cooper from Sencer? Mathews from Cooper? The White House from Mathews? Can a lay policy-maker force some approximation from a reluctant expert? ("You don't need to tell me, I'll tell you. You just let me know if I'm right. Does fifty percent sound too high? . . .")

Probabilities do not create a complete decision analysis, but in 1976 a less-than-complete analysis could still have been illuminating. Probability estimates smoke out differences in expert views which laymen need to see. Discrepancies in expert views underscore the merits of a "hedge" strategy: delay the delayable while probing for more information. Precisely that emphasis was what the actual swine flu decisions lacked from first to last. The lack is readily discovered, its justification readily disputed. The actual decision-making thus becomes a vivid teaching vehicle. Chapters 1–4 convey it, supplemented by 16, while 5–10 deal with outcomes and revisions.

The swine flu program also offers elements of use for teaching quantitative methods in epidemiology. The difficult distinction between influenza-the-virus and influenza-the-disease weakens the epidemiologic data base. This affects everything from studies of vaccine efficacy to detecting the start of an epidemic. Practical issues for epidemiology include tracking the outbreak of disease in a timely way and ascertaining the side effects of immunization.[100] These are prominent in the swine flu case. CDC had five monitoring systems in place to detect influenza: reports of absenteeism from selected industries and schools, and of upper respiratory illness from hospitals; morbidity reports of flu-like illness from physicians in 34 states; anecdotal reports from state epidemiologists; mortality reports from 121 cities; and, in collaboration with the National Center for Health Statistics, reports from the Health Interview Survey, based on weekly interviews at a representative sampling of U.S. households. The teacher can press students to think quite specifically about the usefulness and limitations of each source of information.

As for side effects, associating Guillain-Barré syndrome with swine flu immunization is a notable achievement for surveillance. There was little preexisting information on the epidemiology of Guillain-Barré syndrome; furthermore the syndrome was occasionally hard to diagnose, and worse, not routinely reported. Epidemiology students are asked to detail the investigative steps they would have taken in the face of these obstacles to pin down an association at the time it was first seriously entertained. As investigation actually disclosed in 1976, the incidence of Guillain-Barré syndrome was found to peak two to three weeks after immunization. This time-relation strongly supports an etiologic association. But as a longer time horizon is considered the apparent increase in risk for Guillain-Barré syndrome declines. Over what time-frame should the relative risk be calculated? On what factors should the choice of an end-point depend? How should the results be presented to the public? How should the association influence future immunization programs?

A course on statistical forecasting makes a different use of swine flu. Our report demonstrates the need for more accurate stochastic models of the influenza process—the likelihood of different types of flu, severity of disease in different population groups and regions of the country, and effectiveness of vaccine. The goal is not to determine exactly who will get the flu, but to generate more accurate and precise probability distributions. The teacher asks students to examine recent bases for prediction, including the theories of cycling and recycling, and the time-series model for predicting excess influenza mortality from a five-year moving average of total deaths due to flu and to pneumonia. Combining deaths from influenza and pneumonia produces a more stable and clinically more sensible data base, but one that is less sensitive to changes in the incidence of flu. This illustrates the common tradeoff in statistical analyses between reliability and validity. Students then are asked about additional ways to model the flu process, for example whether and how experience in the Southern Hemisphere can be used to predict flu in the United States. The teacher reviews goals of forecasting in the swine flu affair—which ranged from accurate prediction to behavior change—and spurs discussion of specific, informal methods used, for example in the ACIP deliberations, March 10, 1976. Discussion cannot help but emphasize that forecasting is simultaneously an exercise in statistics and a basis for policy-making.

Institutional Aspects of Policy Analysis

At least one 80-minute class, or equivalent, can be devoted to decision processes at Federal levels in domestic spheres, as illustrated by approvals for the swine flu program during March, 1976. Implicit questions are: who should decide such issues? on what basis? Explicitly, the teacher pushes students up the hierarchical ladder from Sencer to Ford, asking whether each behaved appropriately in the situation thrust upon him. Could Mathews, for example, have arranged the work around him so as to protect himself from Cooper's unchecked thrust? But indeed he had, through Morrill and the General Counsel's office. When they make no resistance must a Mathews do the same? When does the decision come to be inevitable, and for whom? What, if anything, could roll that back? Students are asked to notice questions in the case about the odds of a pandemic and the answers (or non-answers) given, level by level; also the cumulation from one level to the next of certitude about the risk. Could numbers on the probabilities have slowed that? Whose numbers? How get them stated over Cooper's opposition? More broadly, how confront an expert of his temperament? Who does that? (To the student: You?).

A reading assignment to support these questions can be Chapters 1, 16, and the end of 4, together with the text of Sencer's memorandum in Appendix D and Chapter 2 up to the point where he begins to write it. An alternative is Chapters 1–4, along with that memorandum. If time allows, Chapter 6 is usefully read later to put in perspective the initial consensus.

This class can be supplemented by another raising questions on the lines of "thinking about doing" (before doing it) discussed in Chapter 12. The subject, more pretentiously, is "implementation analysis." Unfortunately, to illustrate what might have been foreseen, and how, before the program started—and the limits on such estimates as well as the advantages—there is a need to understand what happened *after* implementation began, in the dimensions of media relations, vaccine testing, liability legislation, slippages of starting dates, contracting, Federal-state-local relations, coincident deaths and side effects. All can be gleaned by reading Chapters 5–11 and appropriate pages in 12, but that becomes a 60-page assignment, which students might not read closely enough for an informed discussion in a single class. The alternative is to pursue but one of those dimensions (incorporating the rest by reference or short lecture), for example media relations. This would require an assignment of no more than 20 pages, culled from the end of Chapters 4 and 6, the start of 7, bits of 8, half of 9 and part of 12 again.

Another classroom use for the material is in conjunction with a closely related subject, "foreign assessment." This means thinking about possible reactions from an outside organization which your actions will affect and which in turn affects your prospects. The swine flu program illustrates one relative success in this respect, relations with the private manufacturers, and one startling failure, non-relations with the casualty insurers. Chapters 6 and 7 give the essence of both stories.

Undergraduate courses in political science afford other, more traditional subjects where the swine flu affair is usefully illustrative. For instance in a course on the American Presidency, where this book as a whole is assigned, it illustrates a lecture on the sorts of personnel—origins, tasks, tenures, incentives, outlooks —that inhabit Federal agencies in modern times, from specialized careerists to generalist appointees and all in between. Thereafter, the swine flu program does double duty in the course as one of several sources repeatedly invoked to illustrate assorted problems and dilemmas faced by modern Presidents, in media, congressional and interest-group relations along with staffing, deadlines and priorities.

Uses of History in Analysis and Management

Eight graduate programs across the country—some of them business schools, some public policy programs, one a law school —are now collaborating in the development of course work on the uses and abuses of historical analogies and other sorts of reference to historical materials which government decision-makers actually employ. The aim is to assess and improve practice, not to deplore it. The theory of the thing, along with teaching notes and cases, will be written up for publication relatively soon.

In this effort the flu program of 1976 serves as a prime example of the power of analogies in policy and also of the limited extent to which the analogues are seriously compared by policy-makers. Failure to compare skews characterization of the problem.

One course under development assigns its students parts of Chapters 1–9 for reading in advance of a two-hour class. Students skim the narrative while concentrating on successive uses of analogies with 1918, 1957 and 1968. The first of these evoked the worldwide killer, the original swine flu, powerfully affecting laymen and doctors alike. The second and third affected mainly the technicians, spurring them to seek a better record sooner than with Asian or Hong Kong flu. To understand these analogues, students also read excerpts from Beveridge, Crosby and Osborn (cited in our Readings). Close comparisons with 1976 are then made during class, by methods devised for the course. Differences show up while likenesses become less overwhelming. This raises questions about other useful analogues and how to search them out. Also it tends to alter characterizations of the problem, hence of what to do in response. Policy implications derived in class are set alongside those chosen by the actual policy-makers. The class then argues whether and to what degree a close look at analogies might have changed any choices during 1976.

Instructors are experimenting with means to ease the load of advance reading for this class. In a lecture course that reading would not be severe but this class depends, as indicated, on informed discussion. Accordingly, we now plan a teaching case to replace, in shorter form, the readings on earlier analogues. If the case seems satisfactory, after trial teaching, it will be made publicly available.

The swine flu report comes up a second time in this same course, along with somewhat comparable documents, to probe the value of vicarious experience imparted by such means to transient officials. The issue is especially provocative for experienced students in executive development programs.

A very different use for this material is in a course on the history of public health. The 1976 swine flu program can be viewed as a benchmark in the evolution of public health programs. In the early decades of this century, mass public health efforts were linked to the waves of immigrants who entered the country, and public health was regarded as a welfare enterprise. Public health officials were reluctant to promise more than they could assuredly deliver. Lacking both a social mandate and reliable means, they shied away from direct disease-control programs. The great pandemic of 1918–1919 provoked public skepticism about the adequacy of social services in general but not doubts about public health professionals. Blocking influenza was not theirs to do and no one thought they could. As better technologies for disease prevention developed, however, these became the medical province and social responsibility of the public health profession. Prominent among these technologies were safe and effective vaccines. The swine flu program marked, at its bold beginning, the most ambitious of immunization ventures, seeking complete coverage within the country. At its hasty close it left behind fresh fears, a heightened cautiousness, a lessened credibility among the laymen and perhaps a lessened confidence among the doctors. It represents at least a temporary peak in this country's public health moves toward direct disease prevention.

Public-Sector Management

Our report to Califano dealt extensively with implementation. This lends itself to classroom use for management courses teaching subjects like indirect management, project management, dealing with experts, and program review.

Indirect management is an extraordinary feature of American public service, especially Federal service. The swine flu story but suggests a rather general situation in which those who actually carry out decisions are neither Federal employees nor otherwise accountable in any direct sense to those who make decisions. Ford could choose to vaccinate the nation and could delegate the doing to Mathews who in turn could delegate to Cooper, hence to Sencer and on down the Federal line. But private laboratories made the vaccine, while a mix of local nurses, city, state or private, stuck it into people who themselves had to turn up, perhaps after consulting their own doctors in the process, or their neighbors, or the newspapers. Ford was a long way from the likes of these and so, it turned out, was the whole of HEW, CDC included.

Once CDC officials grasped a leading role within the Federal government—nominally shared for certain purposes by Cooper's office—how did they try to exercise it with respect to vaccine manufacture, testing, distribution, use, ancillary supplies and personnel, immunization practices, surveillance, contingency plans, later reviews and adjustments? What went right? What wrong? What were the prospects for performance in an actual pandemic? How, if at all, could these have been improved within the web of Federal-state-local and public-private relations? Or could the web have been ignored and direct action substituted, as for instance by using the Army? Under what conditions?

To fuel discussion of these questions, students first read Chapters 5, 6 and 9. Comparable questions could be raised about liability if students also had read Chapters 7 and 8.

Indirect management as manifested here serves readily to introduce the key issue of project management in HEW immediately after Ford announced the swine flu program. "Project management" deals with the ways and means to go after a single, defined goal under time constraints, in this case national immunization before winter. For the balance of an 80-minute class, or in a second class, students can be asked if Cooper was wise to frustrate Mathews' yearnings and Young's scheme for a separate, emergency unit. As a practical matter was Cooper right to lean on the existing, "peacetime" agencies? Were the CDC connections with the states as indispensable to a lead role in the field as Sencer claimed and Cooper evidently thought? One teacher we know, himself a former Undersecretary of HEW, thinks "no" on both scores and he steps out of his role as monitor of student argument to say so at the end of class. But this logically invokes a prior question. Given the personalities and time constraints, along with those connections, how organize effectively the other way? That had been Cooper's question.

Another class can be devoted to a different problem, also illustrated by swine flu, which turns up in public management whenever policy judgment—or administrative feasibility, for that matter—has technical components likely to be veiled from politicians and their generalist advisers. How induce the technicians to explain not only what they know but what they don't in terms evoking managerial judgment from their constitutional superiors (who probably are laymen)? The question runs perhaps as much to spheres of energy, environment, defense, intelligence, diplomacy, economy, as to the sphere of health. Doctors are a special breed of specialist, perhaps, but Cooper's proud refusal to put numbers on subjective probabilities stands as a metaphor for expert reticence in every sphere. What should their superiors do? The question runs to Cooper too when he dealt with experts outside of cardiology. Did he, did Sencer, Dickson, Mathews, OMB and White House aides, in their respective roles as managers or surrogates for same, seek expert judgment appropriately? When doctors balked at numbers on subjective probabilities should laymen have insisted? Might this have made a difference in their actual decisions? Which decisions? What numbers would each student put on the subjective likelihood of every alleged difference? To prepare for arguing these questions students are assigned Chapters 1–3 and 10, along with portions of 4, 6 and 9. (Discussion can be made to dovetail nicely with its counterpart in quantitative methods.)

There is a flip-side to the role of experts in decisions, namely the roles (if any) for both specialized and general publics. In swine flu terms: Who? How? When? Why? Califano's *ad hoc*, televised, advisory-group meeting after the Victoria flu flare-up in Miami seemed to him a model. But for what? Would such exposure have helped earlier? Or hurt? Is it "right," regardless? Are there any legitimate limits?

There remain the issues of program review in managerial terms: how to assure review, when to undertake it, what to do with results. By way of illustration, the first two numbered points in Chapter 12 offer specific proposals. Students can be asked to test the practicality of these against the actual personalities and circumstances during 1976. This calls for reading, in addition to these points, Chapters 3–5 (perhaps adding 15), parts of 6 and 7, the second half of 8, ditto 9. For a contrasting view, students can read Osborn's chapter cited in our Readings.

Key issues to discuss are scheduled reviews and their uses, also triggers for successive steps if indicated by review. Need the purpose of review be predetermined, as in "Alexander's question"? Need a schedule be public? Suppose the manager wants it to happen without saying so? What is his "tickler" system? With respect to triggers, can a President be bothered twice? A Secretary? A Director? And what might be administrative consequences of a given trigger mechanism in such terms as incentives, morale, training, medical consensus, state approvals, congressional relations, media reactions, public support? If students reject our proposals, as they may, what do they offer instead?

Public Health Practice

The swine flu immunization program was an effort to promote the public health, an exercise in preventive medicine. The substance of our report appeals to medical students studying preventive medicine and to public health students, physicians and non-physicians, novices and old hands. They empathize readily with many of the protagonists in the narrative—perhaps they knew some personally. The more experienced students may have worked in the swine flu program and know considerably more about it than we cover. Others just embarking on their professional careers will find most of the case new to them. All students in the field, whatever their professional background, can foresee themselves stuck in a similar fix.

Public health practitioners naturally gravitate to practical questions raised by the case. For example, consider the problem of public acceptance of flu vaccine. Most likely this would still pose a problem today. (A CDC-sponsored survey of public opinion found in 1978 that only 53 percent of Americans would want a flu shot were there to be a national immunization program, the same proportion as in August 1976.) In our swine flu report, public attitudes toward shots, with and without any further outbreaks, are taken to be one of many factors in the doability of the program. The report stresses thinking about these matters prior to the policy decision. But to a public health professional, acceptance of vaccination is not simply a factor to be folded into an implementation estimate. Public reluctance is rather a barrier to be overcome, a challenge to the public health profession. Why don't people take the shots doctors know are good for them? Or wear seat belts, or quit smoking, or get regular exercise, for that matter? What kind of public education is most effective, what incentives work, what ingenious methods have been tried, with what results? The swine flu report prompts these questions, motivates a search for answers. They are large questions, central to the success of many public health ventures, and likely to dog practitioners throughout their careers.

For students in professional degree programs, the swine flu report can enliven discussion of major public health institutions and organizations in the United States. The immunization program was engendered by, and engrafted on, an existing public health system. After reading of the program, students want to learn more about the history, organization and role of the Centers for Disease Control. (The change to "Centers" stems from 1980). Interagency relations, as between CDC, BoB and NIAID, take on more substance than lines on an organization chart.

The swine flu affair lends itself to a discussion of relations between public health officials and private medical practitioners and of the responsibilities and authority of state public health departments vis-à-vis federal agencies. Should state and local officials have had more say in the early formulation of federal policy? If so, by what mechanisms? What is their claim to expertise compared to nationally recognized experts? Would state and local public health officials have been more sensitive to issues of implementation—public acceptance, logistics of administering vaccine, media relations, and so forth? How could private practitioners have been utilized more effectively in the program? What recourse was open to state officials who, as some plainly did, doubted the wisdom of the national program? By the same token, what levers could federal officials use to keep the states in line? These questions raise the issues of indirect management and also of applied ethics discussed elsewhere in this chapter. The state and local public health perspective can be nicely presented through a panel discussion with willing public health officials. It is useful to assign available state documents along with pertinent sections of the GAO Report listed in our Readings.

Physicians and public health workers live professionally with the legacies of the swine flu case. The swine flu report can be an entrée into teaching about larger issues of policy toward immunization and liability.

The swine flu program was one of many vaccination efforts, part of an ongoing struggle against influenza. Students can explore the rationale for current immunization recommendations against flu. Beyond flu, why have some childhood immunization programs, like polio, been so thoroughly successful, while others, like measles, achieved less complete success? What accounts for controversy over the value of some available vaccines, such as pertussis (whooping cough) and pneumococcal (pneumonia) vaccine? What special ethical issues arise when the vaccinee is not the principal target of protection, as in the case of rubella vaccination of youngsters to protect developing fetuses in pregnant women? What is the logic behind public subsidy of some vaccines, but not of others aimed at similar problems (contrast influenza and pneumococcal vaccine)?

What new or heightened problems can be expected from the introduction of many new vaccines currently being tested or developed, such as hepatitis and herpes virus vaccines? As broad-ranging as the swine flu case is, it barely touches on a number of scientific issues about immunization facing public health leaders.

The swine flu program exposed and, for a time, elevated the question of liability for vaccine-related side effects, but the issue was a public health concern well before 1976. Yet it remains unresolved. Vaccine liability ties in to matters of informed consent, of liability for medical research subjects and of general medical liability. These issues make a solution to the liability problem all the more pressing to scientists and public health officials. Students might consider the effect of these related issues on prospects for a Federal, legislative solution. The report from the Congressional Office of Technology Assessment on vaccine-related injuries (listed in our Readings) is a useful background document for classroom discussion of alternative solutions. Should all vaccines be covered? All injuries? If not, what should be the basis for selection? What are the pros and cons of alternative types of compensation and administrative mechanisms? Legally oriented classes can examine the relations between federal legislation and other means of recourse for claims where negligence is not at issue. Public health students and officials also can consider the problem in terms of public advocacy: How could they most effectively press for congressional action? What lessons can be drawn from the effort to get liability legislation in 1976?

The swine flu story can be viewed as policy-making under pressure in a highly technical area. Physicians and public health professionals are, of course, engaged by the technical intricacies of the influenza virus and disease. The technical nature of the issue points to a more general problem: how to obtain expert scientific and technical advice. In research and medicine, as in any technical field, there are gradations of specialization and technical knowledge. There are influenza virologists, general virologists, laboratory scientists, public health generalists, and so forth. Similar hierarchies of specialization could be laid out for immunologists and epidemiologists. Who were the experts in the swine flu problem? Secretary Mathews and President Ford relied on Dr. Cooper for his expert advice. Where does he stand on the hierarchy of expertise? What about Dr. Sencer? What is the proper balance in expert advice between narrow specialization and breadth of view? Who is in a position to judge?

Our swine flu report also stresses the salience of non-scientific, non-medical considerations in formulating and carrying out policy. These are just the analytic and ethical issues covered elsewhere in this chapter. The first four sections of Chapter 12, "Reflections," point to them: building a base for program review, thinking about doing, thinking of the media, and maintaining credibility. To describe these concerns in exclusionary terms, as *non*-scientific and *non*-medical, belittles them in comparison with the scientific, technical issues. They are not less important. The wisdom of any major public health venture depends as much on its rationale in institutional and managerial terms as on its scientific justification. If the teacher can use the swine flu case to sear that lesson into student consciousness, it will have been class time well spent.

We leave to the end of this discussion, although not to the end of our classes, a facet of the swine flu story that is prominent from its outset: the way in which events are inevitably perceived and interpreted according to personal agendas. Sencer, Cooper and others had an abiding faith in the virtue of preventive medicine. Cooper wanted to get the private sector (parents and organizations) firmly committed to public health practices. Stallones saw an opportunity to demonstrate the value of epidemiology to human health. Salk sought the chance to close the immunity gap. Many researchers, also serving as scientific advisers, anticipated an opportunity to learn from the program, regardless of its outcome. Behind these agendas, everyone had vividly in mind the specter of 1918; Meyer, Seal and others also felt keenly the failure to immunize in advance of the epidemics of 1957 and 1968 (see our separate discussion of historical analogues).

We describe these agendas as "personal" because they are individually shaped, tightly held and deeply felt. They are a natural part of the psychology of any dedicated public health official and researcher. They are not mistaken—preventive medicine and public appreciation *are* important, epidemiology *is* underrated, gaps in immunity *do* exist and a great deal *was* learned from the 1976 program—and are only incidentally self-serving. But in concert these agendas riveted attention on an immediate, mass program. The choice emerged from the mind-sets of particular individuals.

We think it is a good thing, on the whole, to become critically aware of the convictions and personal agendas we each bear. By way of prompting self-consciousness, we ask medical and public health students to contemplate the heresy that prevention is not better than cure, at least not always. Many preventives are effective, safe and economical; so are some cures. In some situations, no intervention would be best of all. Any preventive does not, solely by its intent, surpass every other strategic possibility. In the long run, does questioning the wisdom of an unprecedented, mass effort in prevention degrade or reinforce one's advocacy of preventive medicine?

In some cases, could an ounce of do-nothing be worth a pound of prevention?

Ethical Issues in Public Service

Ethical issues manifest themselves to government officials in at least two ways, on the one hand as policy choices in the face of moral codes (is it right to tell the laity only part of the truth?), and on the other hand as conflicts among mutual obligations in relations with associates (is it necessary to speak out against the boss?). The former interest students and will be familiar to them, while the latter seem obscure to pre-careerists.

As an often-taught example from the first of these two categories, the public in a democratic system has a right to question government officials, to know the basis for policy decisions. In the case of immunization, the duty to explain runs deeper, for the success of the policy turns on public understanding. Indeed, programmatic success depends on public *behavior*—people have to line up and get their shots. How should the public official balance the explanation which is most truthful (complete and accurate) against the explanation most likely to assure compliance with the program? Suppose a flare-up of swine flu occurs next year and expert consensus places the risk of pandemic at 5 percent. This is sufficiently great to convince the director of CDC that the public should be immunized. Media and public opinion consultants advise the director to announce "a very real possibility of pandemic" rather than "a one in twenty chance." Their polls suggest that twice as many people would want to get immunized after hearing the former than in recognition of the latter. Having sought explicit probabilities from his advisers, is the director now obliged to lay that 5 percent before the public? Could he avoid doing so, if he wished? Are numbers meaningful to the public anyway? Should risks be couched in more familiar terms (equivalent to the risk of dying in an auto accident, or to getting struck by lightning, etc.)? Within the bounds of truthfulness can he ethically frame the risks to promote public participation? (Warning that there is one chance in 50 of dying may be numerically equivalent to announcing 49 chances in 50 of surviving; psychologically, the former may provoke action, the latter, complacency.) Is the greater obligation to truth or to life? How far can one be sacrificed to serve the other?

Turning to our other category of ethical issues, interpersonal relations, the behavior of a government official on the job is marked by many interpersonal obligations in almost continuous conflict, which nobody resolves for her or him, and indeed no one else can. As citizen he owes a fealty to the country. As official he has sworn an oath to the Constitution. As subordinate he owes at least a formal loyalty up. As superior he owes a loyalty down, and if he cannot give it rarely gets it. He also owes something to his profession, if he has one, and its standards, and he probably adheres to these. As an organization member he owes loyalty to its purposes and to the groups and congressmen that share them. He owes loyalty also to the clientele his organization serves and to its institutional allies in what it does. As purchaser of services he seeks cooperation from his contractors and they from him. If he deals with reporters he evokes their loyalty to a source and they evoke his to an outlet. If his private life is marked by personal interests and attachments, as most are, his loyalties can spread far beyond the job.

And there always are affinities of sex, age, class, ethnicity, religion, education, or the like.

These pull and tug and when they do the government official copes as best he can. The terms on which he does so constitute a large part of the ethical concerns of American public servants. Our swine flu story conveys a whole cross-section of illustrative problems. To name a few: Alexander's discomfiture, Goldfield's outburst—and subsequent chastisement—Sencer's hard sell, Cavanaugh's panel, the leak from the lab, Meriwether's non-job, Hattwick's tunnel-vision, Sabin's June speech, Wecht's pronouncements, Califano's televised treatment of Sencer. Behind each is a complex set of circumstances pitting loyalty against loyalty to produce a necessarily ambiguous result. One can criticize the outcome, but the underlying human calculations are worth sympathetic notice in each case. They underscore how unsimple a thing it is to cope.

They also underscore the absence of sheer villainy. For our report shows none of that. This too we think worth noticing. We also think it is more nearly characteristic of the Federal government than much contemporary commentary holds. However that may be, in this instance there are no evil persons, and not even notably self-interested ones. Everybody's actions turned on trying to pursue the public good. As we were told of Sencer, the most controversial and perhaps most consequential actor in our narrative, he was "a physician with a conscience" trying "to make the strongest case he could."

Moreover, to explain the case in terms of villainy deflects attention from the lessons in a very complicated situation. As good motives do not assure success, evil motives are rarely necessary to explain failure. (Confusion usually suffices.) The swine flu affair may be viewed either as a qualified success or as a qualified failure. We care less about which than about learning from the experience.

To open up these issues in a class we find that Chapter 2 affords the most sharply focused background for discussion: Sencer at CDC, the ACIP meeting, then his action-memorandum. Conflicting obligations have to be resolved; the terms he chooses are perhaps idiosyncratic, but how much so? In the circumstances, as then understood, what might he have weighed differently and so done differently? At what cost to which of his multiple obligations? Should he have paid the cost and altered his behavior? Would this have made his ethical position less ambiguous or more so? In whose eyes?

That last is the ultimate issue. It is hard to be a conscientious doctor and the government's research director in an equal measure all the time. Hard? It proved impossible for Sencer. In the clinch he put the doctor first; we argue that he could and should have done the opposite, playing cool technician rather than driving physician. Had he done so we could raise his ethical score; he probably would lower it.

16

SUB-CABINET

REVIEW

This chapter contains the bulk of a teaching case on swine flu prepared in 1979 for the Kennedy School Case Program at Harvard by J. Bradley O'Connell under the supervision of Professor Laurence E. Lynn, Jr. The case was largely based on research material and notes we had assembled for our 1978 report to Secretary Califano—these we gladly lent—and on the text of the report itself. However, quotations are from interviews separately conducted and subsequently cleared by Messrs. Lynn and O'Connell. Their case, copyrighted by the President and Fellows of Harvard College, is excerpted here with permission.

O'Connell elaborates relations as of 1976 at the assistant-secretary level in HEW, OMB and the White House beyond what we thought necessary for Califano's sake in our original report to him. But for the sake of students we regard the added data as distinctly useful, hence this chapter.

The case begins with the Fort Dix outbreak of January 1976 and continues through the ACIP meeting at CDC on March 10, summarizing chapters 1 and 2 above. Then:

Sencer called Cooper after the meeting and reported that the ACIP unanimously felt the possibility of a major outbreak could not be dismissed and that an extraordinary federal response was probably in order. Sencer added that he and his aides were preparing a more specific memorandum to that effect —in all likelihood recommending a national immunization drive —which he would bring to Washington that weekend. Cooper asked what he called "the usual administrative questions," such as whether CDC had conferred with outside authorities and with the other relevant PHS agencies. Of course, since the actual content of the CDC proposal had not yet been worked out, Cooper did not, at that point, endorse a full-scale immunization drive. Nonetheless, convinced of both the seriousness and urgency of the situation, he believed that some action would be necessary before he returned from the eight-day trip to Egypt on which he was about to depart. Consequently, he took several actions to guarantee that the recommendation Sencer was preparing would receive expeditious consideration. First, so that time would not be lost while the proposal idled in HEW's paper mill, he told Sencer and his own staff to "make sure that Jim Dickson gets it." (James Dickson, the Deputy Assistant Secretary for Health—and like most PHS officials, an M.D.—would be in charge of PHS during Cooper's absence.) Cooper wanted Dickson, in turn, to pass CDC's proposal on to David Mathews, the Secretary of HEW, and see that Sencer had the opportunity to present his case to the Secretary. Cooper also brought the matter up himself, before leaving for Egypt, during one of Mathews' full staff meetings. By Cooper's report, Mathews, who the previous year had left his position as president of the University of Alabama to join the Ford Administration, responded very calmly to the news that the government might have to act rapidly to head off a flu epidemic.

I said that it is my understanding that there may be a need for a recommendation from CDC for a large-scale immunization program in influenza, based on some findings that they are getting from Fort Dix. I said that if that were the case, that would be a rather important discussion, which Dr. Sencer feels needs immediate attention. . . . His reaction was, "Well, we will be pleased to hear it."

He was a rather low-keyed gentleman who wasn't excitable, and there was no great discussion about it that I recall.

Finally, Cooper mentioned to Dr. James Cavanaugh, Deputy Director of the White House staff, that a flu immunization proposal was in the pipeline. A former HEW official, Cavanaugh had, until recently, been Deputy Director of the White House Domestic Council and in charge of the Council's health and welfare staff; he continued to exercise considerable responsibility in these fields for the White House. As Cavanaugh recalled, Cooper said that he felt a full-scale immunization program might be necessary, but that he wanted to be certain first that CDC and the other line health agencies had adequately documented the need for and feasibility of such a program.

Beyond these groundwork-laying activities, Cooper felt no other immediate action at the HEW level (i.e., the Secretary, the Assistant Secretaries and their staff, as opposed to the line agencies) was either necessary or appropriate. In Cooper's estimation, Sencer and CDC were both trustworthy and technically competent; hence, he saw no reason to try to second-guess their conclusions or to reanalyze their raw findings. Moreover, neither his office nor other analysis-and-review operations within the department were set up to undertake that type of medical and epidemiological investigation. As Cooper elaborated:

And what could they evaluate? . . . The evaluation staff wouldn't have a prayer understanding things like that ["jet spread" of an influenza epidemic]. If you want to make government decisions by cross-checking everybody, what you do is set up a long enough lead time that you could set up an evaluation of the proposal, a study time for people to go out and do that. For what was being proposed, that is not a very practical option. . . .

The point is this: if you want to put layers of everything over everything to double-check everybody, then you might as well fire the whole goddamn thing—it ain't worth a damn. The technical expertise is down in the agencies.

Although he did not approve any particular course of action before he left the country, by directing Dickson to go to the

Secretary with Sencer's recommendation, Cooper, in effect, signed off on the general direction Sencer had discussed over the phone.

From March 11–13, Sencer prepared a memorandum bearing the heading "Swine Influenza: ACTION." After the fashion of most government documents, the memo did not bear the name of its author but that of the official at the next higher level of authority; hence, it was written in the form of a recommendation from Cooper to Mathews. [See text, Appendix D.] The seven "Facts" which introduced the paper built the case for a swine flu epidemic in 1976–77 as a serious possibility. Fact #2 was, so to speak, the killer:

The virus isolated at Fort Dix is antigenically related to the influenza virus which has been implicated as the cause of the 1918–19 pandemic which killed 450,000 people—more than 400 out of every 100,000 Americans.

That weekend Sencer arrived in Washington, memo in hand. Since Cooper had made clear that he wanted the recommendation passed on to Mathews, Dickson signed it on his behalf and set up a briefing with the Secretary for Monday morning, March 15. Dickson regarded Sencer as "a very strong man": "It's good to get the strongest man to run something under you—someone who isn't going to destroy the whole operation." He also believed that Sencer's organizational talents had paid off at CDC; he felt Cooper regarded CDC as "a 4+ organization on a 1–4 scale." Perhaps in order to have a counter-balance to Sencer (who was, by some accounts, widely perceived as manipulative as well as well-organized), Dickson invited to the meeting with Mathews the head of another PHS agency, Harry Meyer of the FDA's Bureau of Biologics. Meyer's Bureau would have a crucial role—licensing and testing the vaccine and dealing with the manufacturers—in the event of a "go" decision.

Dickson and Sencer talked very briefly Monday morning and then, along with Meyer, proceeded to the briefing with Mathews. The meeting lasted only about thirty-five minutes but ranged over several topics. Basically repeating the contents of his memo, Sencer took the lead in aggressively advocating a joint public/private program aimed at the entire population, his option #4. Sencer also hinted that Congress (in the person of

Representative Daniel Flood) might act on its own and hold appropriations hearings on swine flu if no immunization initiative emerged from the Department. Mathews' principal question (and the one that most frequently would be posed to *him* over the next ten days) was "What is the probability of an epidemic?" To this, Dickson, Sencer and Meyer unanimously responded, "Unknown." The severity of an epidemic or a pandemic, were it to occur, was also a topic marked by uncertainty, since the virulence of a strain of virus cannot be reliably predicted through laboratory tests. Dickson remarked that the example of 1918–19 served as a "ghastly vignette" to the discussion. Apparently the possibility of one million deaths—an extrapolation, based on the current U.S. population, from the 400,000 deaths of 1918–19—was brought up by someone, despite the fact that today antibiotics could be used during any outbreak;* at any rate, that estimate found its way into a memo later that day from Mathews to the Budget Director.**

Beyond the question of the necessity of a full-scale immunization program was that of its feasibility. As Dickson recalled, they were in a "time-bind"—one of the biggest concerns was chickens, not swine. Flu vaccine is made from killed virus which is grown in eggs. In accordance with the ACIP's January recommendation, the manufacturers had already gone ahead with production of Victoria flu vaccine. Producing swine flu vaccine —on a scale ten times greater than usual—meant making sure the manufacturers could get a whole new batch of eggs; that, in turn, would require above-the-call-of-duty dedication on the part of the chickens.*** Meyer believed that, with some difficulty, it could be done and that vaccine could be ready for distribution by mid-summer. The next major hurdle, also considered "do-able," was to administer the shots before the onset of winter. Sencer thought the program could be completed by sometime in November; Meyer thought "by Christmas" a more realistic estimate.

---

*Although influenza itself is a viral infection, many deaths are caused by bacterial infection on top of the viral pneumonia.

**Other HEW officials recall that the number being "thrown around" most frequently at that time was half a million.

***It was also necessary to act before the food companies made hash out of the roosters as they ordinarily did in the spring.

Although the logistics of the program would be challenging, it was felt certain that a safe and effective vaccine could be developed. Vaccine for other influenza strains had been in use for a quarter of a century, with about 20 million doses administered annually; side effects were anticipated—many arms would be sore and some people would experience fever and chills for a couple of days—but no serious ones. Moreover, two failsafe devices for detecting serious adverse reactions would be put into effect if a program were adopted. First, the Bureau of Biologics would conduct extensive field tests with volunteers before any vaccine was administered to the general population. Second, CDC would set up an elaborate epidemiological surveillance system to monitor both the course of influenza (both swine and Victoria) throughout the season and the incidence of side effects. (Cooper, when he returned, put particular stress on the importance of instituting the surveillance system.)

Meyer did not contradict any of Sencer's hard-sell points but took a more cautious tone. His key caveat to Mathews was that "this is a social and not a scientific decision." All science could do was ascertain that there was a risk of a swine flu pandemic, not how great that risk was. Since criticism could be expected whichever way the Secretary decided, it was important to "bring everybody into the act," to broaden the decision-making beyond the Administration in both the scientific and political communities.

Mathews did not announce a definite decision by the end of the meeting, but judging from the Secretary's reactions, Dickson was convinced that Mathews had concluded it was his responsibility to launch an immunization program. Dickson noted that once officials knew that a pandemic was possible, they could not justify taking no action. Even though the probability of a pandemic (which no one was willing to estimate) could be very low, their concern had to focus on how serious the damage would be if it did occur—and a half million to a million deaths had been mentioned as possible. Dickson commented: "David Mathews was a very sensitive human being and a *historian*. He was not a callous general sending people into battle." He added, "In a political sense, the man didn't exist who could have said 'No.' "

By close of business on Monday, swine flu policymaking outbreaks had occurred in numerous parts of Washington. It was not certain whether HEW would require new authorization legislation in order to launch a swine flu vaccination—that point would have to be explored with its lawyers—but a supplemental appropriation was definitely necessary. That meant that the proposal would have to go through the Executive Office of the President; moreover, getting vaccine production started in time required a more expeditious approach than the usual interagency arrangement for processing requests for supplemental budgets. As Cooper explained the situation:

There is a regular process which is moderately time-consuming . . . regular times when we anticipate the President will consider supplementals. . . . This was outside that time frame. And it would be so unusual we felt that it had to be called specially to his attention.

After the meeting with the PHS officials, Mathews sent a short note to James Lynn, director of the Office of Management and Budget (OMB), inviting him to send someone over to HEW to attend an afternoon briefing on the swine flu threat. The doctors' statements of the uncertainty of a flu outbreak or of its severity somehow did not make it into this memo:

. . . The projections are that this virus will kill one million Americans in 1976. . . . The decision will have to be made in the next week or so. [Full text in Appendix D]

The OMB people were apparently the only officials treated to so strong a statement of the likelihood of a severe epidemic; they also were (and remained) the most doubtful among the federal participants that an outbreak would occur. Even before Mathews formally notified Lynn, OMB staff were working on a swine flu memo of their own. Victor Zafra, chief of the health branch, had read the press accounts in February about the Fort Dix events and the possible return of the 1918–1919 virus; his reaction was "healthy skepticism—I didn't believe them." Around the time of the ACIP meeting, the health staff got word from their HEW counterparts of the probable content of CDC's recommendation. On Saturday, March 13, OMB Deputy Director Paul O'Neill, who was to become the key high-level participant from his agency in the swine flu deliberations, returned to Washington from an out-of-town business trip to find his health staff busy developing their memo:

There were two or three people involved and when I got there they were whirling around the director's office—which includes my office and a couple of secretaries' offices—preparing this memorandum; that's when I first started getting briefed on the issue.

On Monday afternoon, Zafra and his colleagues from OMB, as well as people from the office of Bill Morrill, the HEW Assistant Secretary for Planning and Evaluation, were briefed by the Public Health Service officials (Sencer, Meyer, etc.). Both OMB and Morrill's office pressed the question of probability and were met with the same response Mathews had received— that it was unknown and there was no way of placing a figure on it. Zafra thought that "they hadn't made their case." (He also thought that, in general, the "incentive system" in HEW and in most of the bureaucracy discouraged "asking hard questions," that knocking the conventional wisdom was rewarded only in places like OMB, which incubated skepticism.) Zafra felt a number of aspects of the Fort Dix outbreak suggested that the virus there had neither the spread nor virulence traits of the 1918 disease. First, the outbreak had occurred under unusual circumstances that made people especially susceptible to infectious disease—a crowded living situation and a pool of recruits not yet adjusted to the physical rigors of military life. Second, even under these conditions, only a handful on the entire base had been stricken with swine flu; many others had apparently been exposed but successfully resisted it.* Nonetheless, the tone of the internal OMB memorandum on the subject was cautious. Nancy Bateman, a budget examiner, noted that extensive epidemiological surveillance had turned up no outbreak other than at Fort Dix and also suggested that CDC might have overestimated the budget required for an immunization program.[101] Zafra recalled that OMB staff "did not know

---

*In fact, it later came to light that after the recruit who died of swine flu had collapsed (during a forced march which he had joined against doctors' orders), his sergeant had administered mouth-to-mouth resuscitation, but had not subsequently contracted the disease.

enough to say [a program] was definitely bad." Of course, OMB's reservations (which it tactfully labeled "Uncertainties") did not really puncture HEW's position since Zafra *et al.* could not rule out the possibility of a pandemic.

March 15 also saw greater involvement with the swine flu issue on the part of the White House. At 7:00 that morning Paul O'Neill of OMB brought up the subject over breakfast at the White House with James Cannon, a former Rockefeller aide who was executive director of the Domestic Council in the Ford Administration. Later that morning Cannon and O'Neill mentioned it to President Ford while meeting with him on another subject. In the afternoon, Dr. Dickson called the deputy director of the Domestic Council, James Cavanaugh (whom Cooper had alerted before his departure), and filled him in on the day's events at HEW. Dickson said that Mathews seemed receptive to CDC's immunization proposal and would probably be seeking Executive approval for a supplemental appropriation request very soon. He also transmitted to the White House a copy of Sencer's memorandum. Cavanaugh's reaction to the news was, by Dickson's recollection, characteristically brief and noncommittal: "Okay, Jim, thanks." Dr.* Cavanaugh also had conversations that day with both O'Neill and Mathews during which the topic of swine flu came up. The rest of the week saw further internal consultations and memo-trading within HEW, OMB and the White House; meanwhile, Dickson, O'Neill and Cavanaugh emerged as the principal "trouble-shooters" for their respective departments in anticipation of what they all saw as an inevitable need to involve the President in the decision very soon. The questions being asked all around fell roughly into four categories: probability, production, administration and legal issues. The probability issue was no clearer than it had been on Monday or, for that matter, in the CDC/NIAID/Bureau of Biologics meetings the previous month; it was "between 1 and 99 percent," and that was as close as science could come to an estimate. The production issue came down to the availability of roosters, chickens, and cooperative, efficient manufacturers. The organizational capability of CDC and, ul-

---

*Cavanaugh's doctorate was a Ph.D., not an M.D.

timately, of the state and local health departments to administer twice as many vaccinations in half as much time as the largest previous federal immunization campaign (the Sabin polio vaccine) also required investigation. Finally, was authorizing legislation necessary before undertaking the campaign, and would the program expose the federal government to frivolous or legitimate lawsuits alleging injuries from vaccinations?

At HEW Mathews relied on a number of what he called "defensive secondaries" to detect any gaps in the line agencies' analysis and recommendations in these areas. Bill Morrill, Assistant Secretary for Planning and Evaluation at HEW, commented on Mathews' operating style in cases like this:

David more nearly reacted to than drove the process. He did not view his role, as a general matter, as being involved in the activities that were particular to a given assistant secretary. He was much more a delegator. . . . He'd have his own agenda of things that he was particularly interested in that he was working on.

Morrill was one of the people Mathews turned to for advice. Since this was not the long-range "policy development" type of question that normally concerned his office, Morrill's involvement was more personal than institutional. Lacking time to launch a formal feasibility study of the proposed program, Mathews basically asked Morrill (and subsequently others) if he thought, on the basis of his own administrative experience and the known facts about flu and vaccinations, a full-scale program could be pulled off operationally:

There was not then, or indeed very much later, the kind of official involvement with the Planning and Evaluation offices that pertained to some other issues, because this was more nearly considered an operational matter that was right on top of us. So the involvement was for the most part by me individually and to a somewhat lesser degree a few of my people. . . . But it was, particularly at that stage, a very fast moving set of events.

Morrill's view of the situation, for the most part, coincided with that of PHS; since this was reportedly often not the case, his concurrence probably carried added weight. As Morrill recalled:

There wasn't anything in this particular undertaking other than sheer size that would lead one to think you couldn't do it. The manufacturing capability [was there] if you got it going; there was clearly a timing issue about whether you could get it all done fast enough. The distributional systems were all in place—the volume of stuff was not so large that it was overtaxed. . . . There didn't seem to be any intrinsic flaws.

In much the same way as with Morrill, Mathews turned to Jack Young, the Comptroller of the department, for advice. Since this was, in part, a budgetary matter, Young's office was involved in an official capacity. Nonetheless, Young, like Cooper, Dickson, Mathews, Morrill *et al.*, did not feel he was in a position to second-guess what appeared to be the consensus of scientific opinion. At the end of the week, he responded through a memorandum to Mathews' query:

I concur with Dr. Cooper's recommendation that you adopt a combined approach to the Swine influenza problem as detailed in alternative number 4. In situations such as this, I see no alternative but to rely upon the advice of our health professionals.[102]

In the meantime, HEW Deputy General Counsel St. John Barrett (who was in charge of the Office of General Counsel [OGC] while William H. Taft IV awaited confirmation as the new General Counsel) told Mathews and Dickson that "under existing statutory authority they could go ahead" with a federally sponsored influenza immunization program; HEW would have to go to Congress only with a request for a supplemental appropriation, not authorization legislation as well. A second area of potential legal difficulties was liability. Both the lawyers and non-lawyers in the department were aware that a trend in court decisions over the past several years was to hold manufacturers "strictly liable" for injuries relating to risks inherent in the product even where there was no defect or negligence involved; producers could shield themselves only by informing the consumer beforehand of any risks associated with the product. Another court decision, dealing with the "duty to warn," was also of particular interest to HEW officials, even before the swine flu issue came up. In 1974, in *Reyes* v. *Wyeth*, the court held that although warnings—to the effect that in very rare instances live-virus vaccine could cause polio—were included in the shipping cartons containing the vaccine, the manufacturer was still liable in a case in which this occurred because the warning had not been communicated directly to the vaccine recipient.

Since the manufacturers would be producing swine flu vaccine to government specifications, federal assumption of the "duty to warn" seemed the easiest solution; both Taft and Barrett thought this would assuage any fears on the part of the manufacturers. The federal government, in turn, could protect itself by writing a warning that accurately communicated the risks associated with the vaccine: sore arms, occasional fever symptoms for a day or two and any other adverse reactions revealed by the vaccine field tests. The only unusual legal step anticipated at that point was that OGC, rather than the line agencies, would be responsible for drafting and negotiating the vaccine purchase contracts with the manufacturers; language pertaining to the government's assumption of the duty to warn would be inserted in the contracts. In retrospect, HEW officials felt they were too complacent in believing that no extraordinary measures for handling liability in a massive federally sponsored immunization program were necessary. Barrett remarked: "We were aware of *Reyes* but didn't regard it [liability] as as serious a problem as it later developed to be. . . . We didn't anticipate the extreme sensitivity of the manufacturers regarding their insurance." At that stage, of course, OGC had simply been consulted by Mathews and Dickson and was not in direct contact with the manufacturers. Dickson was in touch with CDC and the Bureau of Biologics, which informed him that the manufacturers indicated they saw no problems with the immunization program as recommended in the Sencer memo.

Mathews' base-touching within his department had not turned up either opposition to a mass immunization program or evidence of any insurmountable operational obstacles. Also, Sencer, at Mathews' and Dickson's behest, had polled by telephone his outside panel, the ACIP, and filled them in on the details of the vaccination proposal and the status of the federal decision-making; Sencer reported back their unanimous concurrence. Although Cooper, the nation's principal health officer, was in Egypt at the time, he remained something of an invisible presence both inside and outside the department. The immunization program was perceived as Cooper's recommendation and Dickson as Cooper's agent. (If anyone had doubts as to whether Cooper strongly endorsed the proposal, these were certainly dispelled when he returned to Washington at the beginning of the next week.) By the end of the week, a consensus of sorts had evolved among the HEW officials. Morrill summarized:

The Secretary sort of polled, and I can remember myself saying, "Yes, I think you can't just sit on this. You've got to do something." Indeed what characterized the whole set of situations is that the people at the top of the department came pretty quickly to a belief that inaction—to take this report that this thing might happen and to do nothing—was simply untenable. . . . And people were mindful of the fact that it was a presidential election year and that made the thing dreadfully more difficult in a sense—the consequences of doing nothing and then having it later come to light.

The seriousness of the swine flu threat—and the fact that its likelihood couldn't be quantified—weighed heavily on the nonmedical officials. A comment of William Taft, the General Counsel, indicates how this matter filtered up to those regions of the department most distant from CDC's epidemiologists: "The chances seemed to be 1 in 2 that swine flu would come." An unknown probability translated into an even bet. Participants agreed that it was very unusual for the HEW bureaucracy to arrive at a common understanding of a problem (and to act on it as well) within only a week's time. Nonetheless, as one reflected:

HEW, with all its lumbering glacial qualities, was and is able under certain kinds of circumstances to move very fast about some things. . . . If there's potential life-threatening things involved, that agency, and indeed most big agencies like that, can move with surprising, lightninglike speed.

At OMB, Victor Zafra remained very skeptical of the likelihood of a swine flu epidemic; he was also not happy that CDC had gone public with its epidemic warnings considerably before the matter had received any Presidential attention. Likewise,

Paul O'Neill was not convinced that there would be a swine flu epidemic, but he did believe that the possibility was serious enough to worry about. According to him, the safety and effectiveness of a vaccine were not considered problem areas by OMB:

I think there was an acceptance of the capability of the scientists. While I don't think it was ever spoken explicitly, there was an assumption that if the immunologists could produce a polio vaccine that could stop the tragedy of polio epidemic, then they certainly would produce a [swine flu] vaccine. They said they could produce a successful vaccine—very quickly and with no problems. There was an acceptance of the notion of scientific credentials.

During the course of swine flu discussions at OMB, an issue resurfaced that had been discussed in Atlanta, both within CDC and in the ACIP meeting, but had not made it into Sencer's memorandum. Could the government order production of vaccine now and agree to purchase enough for the whole population, but hold back on administering it until there was confirmed evidence of an outbreak? The word back from HEW on each occasion (Cavanaugh brought it up also) was that for both logistical and medical reasons there would not be sufficient time. It was estimated that an epidemic could spread throughout a city in about two weeks; because of air travel, it was conceivable that it could spread through the country almost as quickly. PHS contended that it would be impossible to distribute and administer it to all who wanted it in that amount of time—the public health network would be able to manage 200 million vaccinations, but only at a more leisurely pace. Moreover, even if the public and private health practitioners could get the vaccine into people's arms in a few weeks, still more time would be needed before the shots conferred immunity. As Cooper, who upon his return stood with the line agency chiefs in opposing stockpiling, elaborated:

You thought you had a substance that was safe and effective. What you would want to do is get it out early enough because effective immunization at a biologic level requires several weeks to generate the antibody response. So the ideal time to do it would be to get it out and into the folks early and get the antibody response on board. That was the concept of prevention, not a reaction to a thing.

OMB accepted the judgment that stockpiling was not feasible. On budgetary grounds, there was no reason to favor it over the preventive immunization approach; all but $8 million (for administration) of the requested $134 million would go for purchase of the vaccine in either case. Moreover, if stockpiling meant that not everyone who wanted the vaccine could receive it in time, the Administration might be held accountable for the exclusion of some groups. O'Neill recalled:

It seems to me that there was a fairly convincing argument that if the inoculation program didn't begin almost as soon as the vaccine became available that it wouldn't be possible to inoculate the whole population and, therefore, you'd be making the decision that those people who didn't get in because of the time delay were the risk population, that had been put in that position because of the delay in the decision process.

By the end of the week of March 15, the OMB leadership had arrived at much the same perspective as their HEW counterparts. "Ultimately," said O'Neill, "in our judgment—that is to say, mine and Jim Lynn's—the President didn't have much choice." Even Zafra agreed that although an epidemic might be technically unlikely, the government was by this time boxed in: "The President made the necessary political choice." It was also assumed by everyone involved with the issue that the final decision on swine flu immunization had to come from Gerald Ford. Simply as a procedural matter, he would have to sign the request for a supplemental appropriation. More importantly to Lynn and O'Neill, this was a decision on whether or not to launch a major new program with considerable implications for life and safety (the estimate of half a million deaths) as well as policy (setting precedents in federal preventive medicine programming). O'Neill commented:

I guess it never occurred to me that, whoever the President might have been, he wouldn't have been deeply involved in this kind of a question. Because the national policy implications of a threat of a major epidemic are not the kind of thing that, in my judgment, ought to be left to HEW and OMB to decide between themselves.

At the White House, James Cannon and James Cavanaugh were equally certain that the President would have to act shortly. "It was a decision that only a President could make," remarked Cannon. Cavanaugh had some "real questions" about the whole immunization proposal after his initial discussions with Mathews and Dickson on March 15. Cavanaugh felt CDC was "historically a very strong advocacy agency"; he saw his own role as "staying on top of the issue" to be certain that the case was backed up by a firm staff analysis. Therefore, Cannon, Cavanaugh and Spencer Johnson, the health analyst on the Domestic Council staff, undertook a review of their own. This, said Cavanaugh, was the usual White House response when a line agency pressed for a new program and marked it with an "urgent timeframe." "There was no 'rush to judgment.' . . . We'd put the issue on a fast-track for decision but be damned sure we'd gotten a full staff review."

Cavanaugh's questions were basically the same as those being asked at HEW and OMB that week, although a few of his channels of investigation were different. As a former HEW man himself, he maintained that he "knew that department like the back of my hand" and that his contacts reached below the level of assistant secretaries and "down into the bowels of the agencies." The first concern, of course, was whether or not the threat was really serious and the immunization program necessary. Cavanaugh called around and did not turn up any criticism on this score; he did, however, encounter the PHS argument that tying the actual start of the vaccination program to evidence of an outbreak was not feasible because of time considerations. He also called an old HEW associate, Dr. Charles Edwards, a former FDA Commissioner and Assistant Secretary for Health. Edwards' line was the same as that of the current PHS leadership: given the available data, immunization directed at the entire population was the only alternative. In the course of Cannon's and Cavanaugh's inquiries, one potential production obstacle disappeared. The Agriculture Department assured them that there were enough chickens to produce enough eggs to produce enough vaccine doses for the country. On the question of liability, Cavanaugh went directly to Attorney General Edward Levi, who referred him to a staff attorney who basically agreed with the HEW attorneys that the liability issue could be managed by having the federal government assume the "duty to warn." Cavanaugh, nonetheless, remembered having some inkling at that point that perhaps some more drastic form of liability bail-out for the manufacturers, such as indemnification legislation, might be needed; in any event, he apparently did not see this as a prohibitive concern. By the end of the week Cavanaugh was resigned to the swine flu decision: "There was no choice."

At Mathews' request, Cavanaugh scheduled a meeting with President Ford for 11:00 A.M. Monday, March 22. Spencer Johnson of the Domestic Council prepared a briefing document, setting out the data about the flu outbreak and the vaccine plans and including comments from the President's other advisers; OMB also sent over a briefing paper of its own, signed by James Lynn, which contained Zafra's "uncertainties." No one offered any objections to the proposed mass immunization program. Nonetheless, the White House people probably would not have agreed with the attitude expressed at the public health workshop the previous month, that coping with an isolated outbreak of a new virus strain was exciting and "stimulating" rather than a "real chore." They insisted that no politics were involved in their support of the immunization program; they anticipated that, if anything, the program would be a political liability—if swine flu did not spread, the President might be cast in the role of a foolish alarmist. Cavanaugh said, "There were no politics; there was some concern that we'd scare a lot of people." Cannon recalled:

It was going to cost a lot of money and great inconvenience to people, and privately some of the political experts around thought that this might be very damaging to the President because people would have sore arms in October, just before the election. . . . That was never a serious consideration, but someone did raise it as a possibility.

As a way of lessening the potential for political embarrassment, Mathews, and subsequently Cooper, offered to announce the program to the public. The suggestion was basically left up in the air, although Cannon's and Cavanaugh's feeling was that convincing people to line up for flu shots would probably require an exercise of Presidential leadership. In any event, the immediate task was making the decision, not announcing it.

By this time the press, having learned something of the week's swine flu activity in the various federal agencies, renewed its interest in the Fort Dix outbreak, the 1918 analogy, and its policy implications. On Sunday, March 21, the day before the scheduled meeting with Ford, swine flu made its second appearance on the front page of the *New York Times*: "Flu Experts Soon to Rule on Need of New Vaccine." The article described the Fort Dix incident as "a single scream in the night and then silence" and reported (inaccurately), "Apparently no recommendation has yet been sent to F. David Mathews, Secretary of Health, Education and Welfare." Both Drs. Sencer and Meyer, as well as several scientists outside the federal government, were quoted as saying that the U.S. would probably have no choice but to mount a large-scale immunization program, albeit on the basis of little evidence that a pandemic was actually on the way: "It's a choice between gambling with money or gambling with lives," declared Meyer.[103]

On the same day as the *New York Times* article, Dr. Theodore Cooper returned to the United States from Egypt. He had not been in touch with Washington during his trip (although he had arranged with Cavanaugh that he could be contacted through the White House switchboard if absolutely necessary), and was unaware of what had transpired during the week. His first piece of new information on the subject came in the form of a message that greeted him upon his arrival at John F. Kennedy Airport that he was to attend a meeting at the White House at 11:00 the next morning. Cooper was briefed on the status of the issue by Dickson and the rest of his staff early Monday morning, and was satisfied that all the potential pitfalls had been adequately explored during his absence. He concluded that there was no other option in the matter and became a forceful advocate of the position already generally supported by the other federal participants.

I don't remember anyone saying "gun to the head" but I do feel that it was my perception that if anyone at the senior level presented that kind of an option, it is very difficult to say "no"—on the basis of the scientific evidence that was available and no other real data that could be used in counterbalancing it. The only other issues at that point were money and time because the questions of both liability and side effects were allegedly spoken to.

Mathews, Cooper and Dickson proceeded to the meeting with President Ford. James Lynn and Paul O'Neill attended from OMB, and James Cannon, James Cavanaugh, Spencer Johnson and Richard Cheney (Ford's chief of staff) from the White House. The HEW group brought along some large briefing boards graphically depicting the swine flu problem and the proposed remedy; Ford, however, apparently preferred to stick to discussion. Mathews began with a general presentation and deferred to Dr. Cooper, as the government's chief medical official, for a more technical explanation of the subject. The President reportedly maintained a "typical Ford" demeanor—"a conservative, quiet listener," asking a few questions. For the most part, the questions and answers remained the same as the ones that had circulated through the agencies. The probability of an epidemic was unknown: no estimates were offered. Serious side effects were not anticipated—field tests and the extensive influenza and reaction surveillance system would detect any risks. Minor side effects such as sore arms and fevers would be common and might be particularly annoying (and possibly politically relevant) if no epidemic materialized. Production and distribution timetables had been mapped out, demonstrating that the project was feasible. Finally, liability concerns had been explored with the government's lawyers, and the line health agencies had reported no dissent on this score from the manufacturers. Mathews added that he knew the program could pose political problems—it was a "no-win situation" for the President whichever way he decided—and repeated his offer that he or Dr. Cooper could take responsibility for publicly announcing it.

There was no devil's advocate *per se* at the meeting; nonetheless, the OMB officials—although convinced by this time that, barring some unexpected development, the government would have to go ahead with a program—remained disturbed by HEW's refusal or inability to give a numerical probability for a pandemic, and hesitant about the program's feasibility. Cooper commented: "They were very leery. They were the most cautious of the group—on very sound and good grounds. They pushed for more broad scientific input." On this issue, the breadth of the scientific review, O'Neill struck a chord with the President. Ford asked, "How wide has the consultation been?" Cooper explained that CDC had followed the usual process of consulting with the other federal health agencies and putting the issue before its standing advisory panel, the ACIP, before bringing it to the level of the HEW secretariat—i.e., no new scientific review body had been set up for the special purpose of studying swine flu. O'Neill argued that such a review should take place at the Presidential level; this was a final opportunity to ferret out any scientific objections to the proposal that had not been raised in HEW as well as a way of extending the decision-making beyond the bureaucracy and the Administration:

I felt very strongly that the President ought to hear from the outside people, and that we ought to marshal people who were—and who would be perceived to be—the leaders in immunology and virology from around the country, so that he had the value of advice from that independent source.

Ford apparently was enthusiastic about the idea of touching base directly with the "scientific community," and asked his aides to assemble a group of experts to meet with him in two days; a conference was scheduled for the afternoon of Wednesday, March 24. Ford deferred his final decision on swine flu immunization until then and did not indicate explicitly what his preferences were; nonetheless, the participants emerged from the Monday meeting with the feeling that the mass vaccination program was now a near-certainty. As James Cannon recounted:

On the basis of the information we had at that time, it would have been in my judgment then, and in my retrospective view, absolutely criminal not to proceed to protect the public health—whatever the political consequences. . . . There was literally time to save what we could extrapolate to be several hundred thousand lives. . . . There was just no question about it.

At the same time, Cavanaugh and Cannon were convinced of the President's sincerity in getting a "spectrum" of scientific opinion and felt that their own role was to make certain he was exposed to any contrary viewpoints before he decided. Cavanaugh had the central task of putting together the "blue-ribbon" panel to meet with Ford. Most of the doctors and scientists he invited were drawn from a list submitted by Cooper, which he in turn had compiled primarily from the suggestions of Sencer and the other line agency heads; Cavanaugh also placed another call to Dr. Edwards, the former Assistant Secretary for Health, who suggested a few more names. Cavanaugh ultimately lined up about thirty non-government scientists for the meeting. The group included several people—such as Maurice Hilleman of Merck, Sharpe and Dohme, Reuel Stallones of the University of Texas, and Edwin Kilbourne of Mt. Sinai Medical School—who had participated in either the Bethesda workshop or the Atlanta ACIP meeting. Officials of other pharmaceutical companies, state and local health departments, and the national medical associations were also invited, along with other sundry guests such as the mayor of Louisville, Kentucky (who happened to be an M.D.), and the Governor of Rhode Island.

The real "coup," from the point of view of the White House, was Cavanaugh's success in securing the attendance of both Dr. Jonas Salk and Dr. Albert Sabin, developers respectively of the killed- and live-virus polio vaccines. To the public their names were probably synonymous with vaccinations. Moreover, it was no secret in the scientific community that there was little love lost between the two "pioneers" in virology, and they tended to square off against one another on most scientific issues. Possibly, Cavanaugh and the others at the White House saw the Salk-Sabin pairing as a final test; if there were faults in the proposal, one of them would be likely to find them. In any event, bringing Salk and Sabin into the decision was considered sufficiently important that the White House brought the latter up to Washington by military jet so that he would not have to bow out of the meeting with the President because of his commitment to address the South Carolina legislature earlier that day. Finally, the federal government would be represented at the meeting by President Ford and most of his staff, Lynn and

O'Neill, and a large delegation from HEW: Mathews, Cooper, Dickson, Sencer, Meyer and the heads of the FDA, the National Institutes of Health and NIAID. No one from Capitol Hill was invited; to the White House aides, including Congressmen would be a political—not a bi-partisan—act. Said Cavanaugh, "These were scientific factual issues, not political ones." In retrospect, the organizers of the panel of experts saw only one serious omission. Cooper commented: "There was nobody there from the insurance industry. Perhaps that is a lesson for something of that order."

The various federal officials recalled this as *the* crucial meeting in swine flu decision-making. Nonetheless, the White House and PHS were sufficiently certain that the March 24 meeting would produce a "go ahead" decision that they set in motion ahead of time the machinery for announcing the program. Earlier in the day, Jim Cannon sent Max Friedersdorf, the congressional liaison aide, a short memo concerning notification of the members of the House and Senate health authorization and appropriations subcommittees. Cannon explained:

The President will brief the press at the conclusion of the meeting to announce his decision to give the go-ahead to pharmaceutical manufacturers to produce enough vaccine to immunize every American, at least 200 million doses.[104]

Also, the PHS and White House press offices stood ready with swine flu "Fact Sheets" ("embargoed for release" until 5:00 P.M.) bearing the same message:

The President . . . is asking Congress to appropriate $135 million prior to their April recess to ensure the production of enough vaccine to inoculate every man, woman and child in the United States.[105]

The feeling of the White House aides was that only in the case of a serious negative response from some of the scientists, which on the basis of their advance checking they saw no reason to expect, would a mass immunization program not be announced officially later that day.

[The case concludes with a summary of the meeting and the subsequent press conference, as described above in chapter 4.]

READINGS:

A SELECTION

W. I. B. Beveridge, *Influenza: The Last Great Plague*, Heinemann, London, 1977.
  Concise, non-technical account of the epidemic behavior of influenza.

Comptroller General of the United States, *The Swine Flu Program: An Unprecedented Venture in Preventive Medicine*, Report to the Congress, June 27, 1977.
  Reviews planning and operation of the swine flu program and offers recommendations.

Alfred W. Crosby, Jr., *Epidemic and Peace, 1918*, Greenwood Press, Westport, Connecticut, 1976.
  Comprehensive, non-technical account of the great influenza pandemic of 1918–19.

The Journal of Infectious Diseases, Volume 136, Supplement, December 1977.
  Reports presented at a symposium sponsored by NIAID, BoB and CDC in January 1977. Introductory papers contain detailed accounts of investigations surrounding identification of swine flu in New Jersey; others deal with clinical studies of swine influenza vaccine.

Edwin D. Kilbourne (editor), *The Influenza Viruses and Influenza*, Academic Press, New York, 1975.

Excellent, authoritative textbook.

Office of Technology Assessment, Congress of the United States, "Compensation for Vaccine-Related Injuries: A Technical Memorandum," Washington, D.C., November 1980.

Assumes some form of a federal compensation program is desirable and discusses issues the Congress will need to consider in adopting legislation.

June Osborn (editor), *Influenza in America 1918–1976*, Prodist, New York, 1977.

Based on a symposium concerning the history, science and politics of influenza held at a meeting of the American Association for the History of Medicine in May 1977.

Philip Selby (editor), *Influenza: Virus, Vaccine and Strategy*, Academic Press, London, 1976.

Papers presented at a conference on pandemic influenza in January 1976; the state of expert thinking just prior to isolation of swine flu in New Jersey.

Sir Charles H. Stuart-Harris and Geoffrey C. Schild, *Influenza: The Viruses and the Disease*, Publishing Sciences Group, Littleton, Massachusetts, 1976.

Technical but well-written summary of knowledge in the field.

United States Senate, *Hearings*, Subcommittee on Health, Committee on Labor and Public Welfare, Ninety-fourth Congress, Second Session, April 1 and August 5, 1976.

Contemporary introduction to the swine flu program's logic and intentions. The August hearing deals with liability.

House of Representatives, *Supplemental Hearings*, Subcommittee on Health and the Environment, Committee on Interstate and Foreign Commerce, Ninety-fourth Congress, Second Session, Serial No. 94–113, June 28, July 20, 23 and September 13, 1976.

Wide-ranging discussion of the swine flu program; emphasizes liability issues. Detail on positions of drug and insurance firms as well as public officials.

NOTES

1. For discussion of influenza types see the Technical Afterword.
2. *New York Times*, February 13, 1976, p. 33, col. 1.
3. Nic Masurel and William M. Marine, "Recycling of Asian and Hong Kong Influenza A Virus Hemagglutinins in Man," *American Journal of Epidemiology* Vol. 97, pp. 48–49, 1973.
4. Some weeks later some of them anonymously contributed their privately held numerical probabilities to an academic study that applied a particular analytic technique, the so-called "Delphi" method, to the swine flu decision. Other experts also contributed numbers anonymously. See Stephen Schoenbaum, Barbara McNeil, and Joel Kavet, "The Swine Influenza Decision," *New England Journal of Medicine*, Vol. 295, pp. 759–765, 1976.
5. For further information on the point, see the report of the General Accounting Office, *The Swine Flu Program: An Unprecedented Venture in Preventive Medicine*, June 27, 1977, Chapter 5; see also Joel Kavet, "Vaccine utilization: trends in the implementation of public policy in the USA," in Philip Selby (editor), *Influenza: Virus, Vaccine and Strategy*, Academic Press, New York and London, 1976, pp. 297–308.

6. Bureau of Biologics Workshop, March 25, 1976, Transcript, p. 128.

7. Here and elsewhere we cite CBS coverage rather than that of NBC or ABC, where all reported the same happening, because only CBS retains transcripts of news stories as telecast or broadcast.

8. Officials of the Health Ministry in Ottawa told us that they had served as a "procurement agent" for the Provinces. As such they tried and failed to get vaccine from U.S. manufacturers; Washington took too long to release it for their use. They contracted eventually with firms in Britain, Germany, Australia and the Netherlands. (These new and multiple suppliers created special testing problems.) Obtaining vaccine only in October, the Canadians suspended shots when we did and like us still have abundant supplies of unused vaccine.

9. Transcript of CBS Evening News, June 22, 1976.

10. Minutes of ACIP-BoB Advisory Panels Meeting, June 22, 1976.

11. Transcript of CBS Evening News, June 22, 1976.

12. Letter from John J. Horan, President, Merck and Company (parent of Merck, Sharpe & Dohme, the vaccine manufacturer), to Secretary Mathews, HEW, April 13, 1976. Comparable letters went to seven senators, four congressmen, two members of the White House staff and three of Mathews' associates. The full paragraph in Horan's letter reporting what he had been told by his primary insurer (Federal Insurance Co., Chubb Corporation group) is as follows:

> Our own insurance carrier has just told us that it is willing to insure us only against negligence or fault on our part. Moreover, because of the massive number of people involved, the carrier considers it not feasible to place any broader coverage in the existing world insurance markets at virtually any price. Thus, the carrier is willing to provide us with protection only against claims arising from our own negligence or failure to manufacture in accordance with government specifications, i.e., against those risks which are clearly our responsibility.

13. Secretary Mathews' press conference, HEW, Washington, July 13, 1976.

14. House of Representatives, Committee on Interstate and Foreign Commerce, Subcommittee on Health and the Environment, *Supplemental Hearings*, 94th Congress, 2nd Session, Serial No. 94–113, June 28, 1976, p. 19.

15. *Ibid.*, July 20, 1976, p. 208.

16. *Weekly Compilation of Presidential Documents*, Vol. 12, No. 30, July 19, 1976, p. 1180.

17. *Ibid.*, Vol. 12, No. 32, August 6, 1976, p. 1249.

18. See House of Representatives, Committee on Interstate and Foreign Commerce, Subcommittee on Health and the Environment, *Supplemental Hearings*, Serial No. 94–113, September 13, 1976, pp. 311–313.

19. The President made this comment September 2 to his Press Secretary who released it to the UPI wire service where it appeared. It was quoted by Marilyn Berger on NBC News that night.

20. Transcript, CBS Morning News, October 13, 1976.

21. Transcript, CBS Evening News, October 13, 1976.

22. *Ibid.*

23. Vanderbilt Television News Archives Index and Abstracts, NBC Evening News, October 13, 1976. The scientist quoted is J. Anthony Morris, who had been discharged in July 1976 from BoB after a long proceeding involving his performance of research there. From then on he maintained that he had been fired in retaliation for his criticism of influenza vaccines and immunizations, up to and including swine flu. FDA officials vehemently deny the charge. The Civil Service Commission has since upheld their action. Morris continues his warnings.

24. Transcript, CBS Radio Archives, October 14, 1976.

25. Transcript, CBS Evening News, October 14, 1976.

26. Figures are taken from unpublished data compiled by the CDC. Percentages are based on populations 18 years of age and older, as of the 1970 census. This means that for 1976, percentages are overstated in areas of recent, rapid growth.

27. For full text see HEW press release, December 16, 1976.

28. Memorandum from the Secretary of HEW to the President, "Outbreak of A-Victoria and Formation of Ad Hoc Committee," February 4, 1977.

29. *Washington Post*, February 8, 1977, p. A2, Col. 1, continuation of article entitled "Limited Flu Shot Plan Urged" by Victor Cohn, p. A1, Col. 6.

30. *New York Times*, February 10, 1977, p. 38, Col. 1, editorial entitled, "The Califano Prescription for Flu."

31. *Washington Post*, February 13, 1977, p. C6, Col. 1, editorial entitled, "Swine Flu: Letting the Sunshine In."

32. United States Senate, Committee on Labor and Public Welfare, Subcommittee on Health, *Hearings*, September 23, 1976, p. 57.

33. Office of Assistant Secretary for Health, Contract 263-77-e-0076, *Reports and Recommendations of the National Immunization Work Groups*, "Research and Development," March 11, 1977, p. 4.

34. The trivalent vaccine recommended for use during the winter of 1978–79 was to include first, vaccine against Russian flu; second, vaccine against Victoria or Texas flu, and third, vaccine against the prevailing strain of mild, type-B virus. For discussions of nomenclature see the Technical Afterword.

35. See note 4.

36. In 1976 Carballo was human resources Secretary in the State of Wisconsin; Goldmark, who had held a comparable post in Massachusetts, was Director of the New York State Budget; Stevens was Goldmark's successor in Massachusetts as Secretary for Human Resources.

37. In the course of this study we screened tapes and read summaries of all relevant evening news shows on all three networks from February 1976 through March 1977. Tapes and summaries were made available by Vanderbilt University. We also read applicable transcripts of all CBS News coverage, evening, morning and radio. These came to us courtesy of CBS News. For press and magazine coverage we used clippings compiled contemporaneously for CDC. We subsequently interviewed reporters and others in both types of media.

Another view of coverage in the media is offered by David M. Rubin, "Remember Swine-flu?" *Columbia Journalism Review*, July/August 1977. Surveying samples of TV and press coverage for the week of excitement over temporally related deaths in Pittsburgh (October 11–17, 1976), Professor Rubin finds reporting generally ". . . neither sensational nor inaccurate. On the contrary it faithfully reflected the confusion among public officials. . . ." This squares with our impression throughout the 13 months. Rubin is concerned for the profession of journalism. (He trains journalists at NYU.) He wishes *his* professionals had done much better than they did. We who train public servants feel we have to take the journalism "as is." For what it is worth, we think the swine flu coverage rather better than average. *Our* concern is with that confusion among officials.

Rubin has also put his findings before doctors with suggestions to improve performance in their profession. See David M. Rubin and Val Hendy, "Swine Influenza and the News Media," *Annals of Internal Medicine*, Vol. 87, pp. 769–774, 1977.

38. For that matter, why stop with Federal programs? Deciding proper boundaries for a competition raises issues about Federal-state and public-private roles. This is one reason why such boundaries don't get set. Consider, for example, pneumococcal pneumonia, a frequent cause of death for aged persons and for others at high risk, including persons—many of them children—whose spleens have been removed after an accident. A newly marketed vaccine reliably prevents infection from the 14 common subtypes of the pneumococcus. These account for 80 percent of this pneumonia. The preventive is apparently both safe and lasting. It could prolong thousands of lives each year. The disease is not highly communicable, but it is far more serious for most of those who get it than is influenza. Does this argue for a Federal initiative? If so, at the expense of the flu program? We pose these questions not to answer them but to suggest the range of readily conceivable budgetary tradeoffs. As this shows, however, a competitive arena is not easily established. In the case of influenza, none yet exists.

39. Sir Charles H. Stuart-Harris and Geoffrey C. Schild, *Influenza: The Viruses and the Disease*, Publishing Sciences Group, Inc., Littleton, MA, 1976, pp. 96–111.

40. Chien Liu, "Influenza." Ch. 27 in Paul C. Hoeprich (editor), *Infectious Diseases*, Harper and Row, 1977, pp. 271–276.

41. J. Housworth and A. D. Langmuir, "Excess mortality from epidemic influenza, 1957–1966," *American Journal of Epidemiology*, Vol. 100, pp. 40–48, 1974. See also S. D. Collins,

"Excess Deaths from Pneumonia and Influenza and from Important Chronic Diseases During Epidemics, 1918–1951," United States Public Health Service, *Public Health Monograph No. 10*, U.S. Government Printing Office, Washington, D.C. 1952, pp. 6–7.

42. Robert E. Serfling, "Methods for Current Statistical Analysis of Excess Pneumonia-Influenza Deaths," *Public Health Reports*, Vol. 78, No. 6, June, 1963, pp. 494–506.

43. T. C. Eickhoff, I. L. Sherman and R. E. Serfling, "Observations on excess mortality associated with epidemic influenza," *Journal of the American Medical Association*, Vol. 176, pp. 776–782, 1961.

44. Albert B. Sabin, "Mortality from Pneumonia and Risk Conditions During Influenza Epidemics: high influenza morbidity during non-pandemic years," *Journal of the American Medical Association*, Vol. 237, pp. 2823–2828, 1977. Epidemiologists from CDC published a response to Sabin's article criticizing his methodology, but acknowledging that CDC excess mortality estimates are likely to differ from those based on NCHS mortality data for the entire country. See Michael B. Gregg, Dennis J. Bregman, Richard J. O'Brien, J. Donald Millar, "Influenza Related Mortality," *Journal of the American Medical Association*, Vol. 239, pp. 115–116, 1978.

45. See, for example, Marc Lalonde, *Hospital Morbidity and Total Mortality in Canada*, Canadian Department of Health and Welfare, Long-range Planning Branch, Health Programs Branch, Ottawa, Ontario, October 1973.

46. These are published as a series by the National Center for Health Statistics. See, for example, "Current Estimates from the Health Interview Survey, United States—1974," Vital and Health Statistics, Series 10—No. 100, DHEW Publication No. (HRA) 76–1527, September, 1975.

47. C. H. Stuart-Harris, G. C. Schild, *op. cit.*, pp. 38–39.

48. *Ibid.*, pp. 57–68.

49. This designation indicates a Type A influenza virus first isolated from man in New Jersey in 1976. It contains Hsw1 hemagglutinin (first identified in virus isolated from swine) and N1 neuraminidase.

50. W. I. B. Beveridge, *Influenza: The Last Great Plague*. Heinemann, London, 1977, p. 9.

51. C. H. Stuart-Harris, G. C. Schild, *op. cit.*, pp. 146–148.

52. W. I. B. Beveridge, *op cit.*, p. 33.

53. Epidemic influenza has a predilection for winter, yet most pandemics have begun outside the winter months. *Ibid.*, p. 46.

54. *Ibid.*, pp. 34–35.

55. *Ibid.*, pp. 24–38.

56. The theory was first espoused by Nic Masurel and William M. Marine, "Recycling of Asian and Hong Kong Influenza A Virus Hemagglutinins in Man," *American Journal of Epidemiology*, Vol. 97, pp. 44–49, 1973.

57. S. C. Schoenbaum, M. T. Coleman, W. R. Dowdle and S. R. Mostow, "Epidemiology of Influenza in the Elderly: Evidence of Virus Recycling," *American Journal of Epidemiology*, Vol. 103, pp. 166–173, 1976.

58. C. H. Stuart-Harris, G. C. Schild, *op. cit.*, pp. 62–68.

59. W. I. B. Beveridge, *op. cit.*, p. 78. See also W. R. Dowdle, "Approaches to the Control of Pandemic Influenza," International Conference on the Application of Vaccines Against Viral, Rickettsial, and Bacterial Diseases of Man, Washington, D.C., 14–18 December 1970, pp. 86–87.

60. The 1950 virus was a further minor drift; it now has reappeared as Russian flu.

61. W. R. Dowdle, "Influenza: Epidemic Patterns and Antigenic Variation," in Philip Selby (editor), *Influenza: Virus, Vaccine and Strategy*, Academic Press, New York and London, 1976, pp. 17–21.

62. See, for example, J. Kavet, "A Perspective on the Significance of Pandemic Influenza," *American Journal of Public Health*, Vol. 67, pp. 1063–1070, 1977.

63. "Amantadine for High-risk Influenza," *The Medical Letter*, Vol. 20, No. 5 (Issue 500), March 10, 1978.

64. G. F. Jackson, "Sensitivity of Influenza A Virus to Amantadine," *Journal of Infectious Diseases*, Vol. 136, pp. 301–302, 1972. See also A. Chanin, "Influenza: Vaccines or Amantadine," *Journal of the American Medical Association*, Vol. 237, p. 1445, 1977.

65. Chien Liu, *op. cit.*, p. 275.

66. C. H. Stuart-Harris, G. C. Schild, *op. cit.*, p. 203.

67. *Ibid.*, p. 164.

68. *Ibid.*, p. 150.

69. J. Salk and D. Salk, "Control of Influenza and Poliomyelitis With Killed Virus Vaccines," *Science*, Vol. 195, 4 March 1977, p. 842.

70. J. W. F. Smith, "Vaccination Strategy," in P. Selby, *op. cit.*, pp. 277–78.

71. *Ibid.*, p. 278.

72. C. H. Stuart-Harris, G. C. Schild, *op. cit.*, pp. 185–193.

73. D. A. J. Tyrrell, "Inactivated Whole Virus Vaccine," in P. Selby, *op. cit.*, pp. 137–140.

74. E. D. Kilbourne, "Future Influenza Vaccines and the Use of Genetic Recombinants," *Bulletin of the World Health Organization*, Vol. 41, 1969, p. 643.

75. H. B. Dull and W. R. Dowdle, "Influenza," in P. E. Sartwell (editor), *Marcy-Roseman's Preventive Medicine and Public Health*, 10th ed., Appleton-Century-Crofts, New York, 1973, p. 74.

76. W. I. B. Beveridge, *op. cit.*, p. 95.

77. J. W. F. Smith, "Vaccination Strategy," in P. Selby, *op. cit.*, p. 280.

78. C. H. Stuart-Harris, G. C. Schild, *op. cit.*, pp. 148–159.

79. H. B. Dull and W. R. Dowdle, "Influenza," in P. E. Sartwell, *op. cit.*, p. 72.

80. C. H. Stuart-Harris, G. C. Schild, *op. cit.*, 175–176.

81. Congressional Record, August 4, 1978, Vol. 124, No. 121, p. S.12585.

82. See Joseph A. Califano, Jr., *Governing America: An Insider's Report from the White House and the Cabinet*, New York: Simon & Schuster, 1981, p. 178.

83. "Follow-up on Respiratory Illness—Philadelphia," *Morbidity and Mortality Weekly Reports*, Vol. 26, No. 2, pp. 9–11, January 18, 1977. "Follow-up on Toxic Shock Syndrome—United States," *Morbidity and Mortality Weekly Reports*, Vol. 29, No. 25, pp. 297–299, June 27, 1980.

84. U.S. Congress, Office of Technology Assessment, "Compensation for Vaccine-Related Injuries: A Technical Memorandum," Washington, D.C., November 1980.

85. See J. A. Califano, *op. cit.*, p. 179.

86. M. Getling, J. Bye, J. Skehel and M. Waterfield, "Cloning and DNA Sequence of Double-Stranded Copies of Haemagglutinin

Genes from H2 and H3 Strains Elucidate Antigenic Shift and Drift in Human Influenza Virus," *Nature*, Vol. 287, pp. 301–306, 1980. M. Verhoyen, R. Fang, W. M. Jou, R. Devos, D. Huylebroeck, E. Saman and W. Fiers, "Antigenic Drift Between the Haemagglutinin of the Hong Kong Influenza Strains A/Aichi/2/68 and A/Victoria/3/75," *Nature*, Vol. 286, pp. 771–776, 1980. S. Fields, G. Winter and G. G. Brownlee, "Structure of the Neuraminidase Gene in Human Influenza Virus A/PR/8/34," *Nature*, Vol. 290, pp. 213–217, 1981.

87. I. A. Wilson, J. J. Skehel, and D. C. Wiley, "Structure of the Haemagglutinin Membrane Glycoprotein of Influenza Virus at 3 Å Resolution," *Nature*, Vol. 289, pp. 366–373, 1981. D. C. Wiley, I. A. Wilson, and J. J. Skehel, "Structural Identification of the Antibody-Binding Sites of Hong Kong Influenza Haemagglutinin and their Involvement in Antigenic Variation," *Nature*, Vol. 289, pp. 373–379, 1981.

88. R. A. Lamb, P. W. Choppin, R. M. Chanock, and G. Lai, "Mapping of the Two Overlapping Genes for Polypeptides NS_1 and NS_2 on RNA Segment 8 of Influenza Virus Genome," *Proceedings of the National Academy of Sciences, U.S.A.*, Vol. 77, pp. 1857–1861, 1980. W. Gerhard, J. Yewdell, M. E. Frankel, and R. Webster, "Antigenic Structure of Influenza Virus Haemagglutinin Defined by Hybridoma Antibodies," *Nature*, Vol. 290, pp. 713–716, 1981.

89. Centers for Disease Control, "Influenza Vaccine 1980–81," *Morbidity and Mortality Weekly Reports*, Vol. 29, No. 19, pp. 225–228, May 16, 1980.

90. W. B. Baine, J. T. Luby, and S. M. Martin, "Severe Illness with Influenza B," *American Journal of Medicine*, Vol. 68, pp. 181–189, 1980.

91. Centers for Disease Control, "Influenza—United States, Worldwide," *Morbidity and Mortality Weekly Reports*, Vol. 29, No. 40, p. 504, October 17, 1980.

92. "Amantadine: Does It Have a Role in the Prevention and Treatment of Influenza?" National Institutes of Health Consensus Development Conference, Oct. 15–16, 1979, *Annals of Internal Medicine*, Vol. 92, pp. 256–258, 1980. See also T. H. Maugh II, "Panel Urges Wide Use of Antiviral Drug," *Science*, Vol. 206, pp. 1058–1060, 1979.

93. F. A. Ennis, R. E. Mayner, D. W. Barry, J. E. Maruschewitz, R. C. Dunlop, and G. C. Schild, "Correlation of Laboratory Studies with Clinical Responses to A/New Jersey Influenza Vaccines," *The Journal of Infectious Diseases*, Vol. 136 (supplement), pp. S397–406, 1977.

94. H. M. Foy, I. Allan, J. M. Blumhagen, M. K. Cooney, C. Hall, and J. P. Fox, "A/USSR and B/Hong Kong Vaccine: Field Experiences During an A/Brazil and an Influenza B Epidemic," *Journal of the American Medical Association*, Vol. 245, pp. 1736–1740, 1981. T. W. Haskins, J. Davies, A. J. Smith, C. Miller, and A. Allchin, "Assessment of Inactivated Influenza-A Vaccine after Three Outbreaks of Influenza A at Christ's Hospital," *Lancet*, Vol. i, pp. 33–35, 1979.

95. T. F. Nolan, Jr., "Influenza Vaccine Efficacy," *Journal of the American Medical Association*, Vol. 245, p. 1762, 1981.

96. Centers for Disease Control, "Influenza Vaccine 1981–82," *Morbidity and Mortality Weekly Reports*, Vol. 30, No, 23, pp. 279–282, 287–288, June 19, 1981.

97. E. S. Hurwitz, L. B. Schonberger, D. B. Nelson, and R. C. Holman, "Guillain-Barré Syndrome and the 1978–1979 Influenza Vaccine," *New England Journal of Medicine*, Vol. 304, pp. 1557–1561, 1981.

98. J. S. Marks and T. J. Halpin, "Guillain-Barré Syndrome in Recipients of A/New Jersey Influenza Vaccine," *Journal of the American Medical Association*, Vol. 243, pp. 2490–2494, 1980.

99. One analysis from an economic, social policy perspective appeared during the swine flu immunization program in the fall of 1976: S. C. Schoenbaum, B. J. McNeil, and J. Kavet, "The Swine-Influenza Decision," *New England Journal of Medicine*, Vol. 295, pp. 759–765, 1976. Another decision analysis from an individual perspective was published more recently: D. L. Zalkind and R. H. Shachtman, "A Decision Analysis Approach to the Swine Influenza Vaccination Decision for an Individual," *Medical Care*, Vol. XVIII, pp. 59–72, 1980.

100. The rapid reporting system for influenza that was developed by the National Center for Health Statistics is described by G. S. Poe and J. T. Massey, "Estimating Influenza Cases and Vaccinations by Means of Weekly Rapid Reporting System,"

Public Health Reports, Vol. 92, pp. 299–306, 1977. A detailed investigation of the association between Guillain-Barré syndrome and swine flu vaccination in Ohio is reported by J. S. Marks and T. J. Halpin, "Guillain-Barré Syndrome in Recipients of A/New Jersey Influenza Vaccine," *Journal of the American Medical Association*, Vol. 243, pp. 2490–2494, 1980.

101. Memorandum from Nancy Bateman, Budget Examiner, to Paul O'Neill, Deputy Director of OMB, March 15, 1976.

102. Memorandum from John Young, Comptroller of HEW, to Secretary Mathews, March 18, 1976.

103. Harold Schmeck, "Flu Experts Soon to Rule on Need of New Vaccine," *New York Times*, pp. 1, 39.

104. Memorandum from James Cannon to Max Friedersdorf, March 24, 1976.

105. Office of the White House Press Secretary, Fact Sheet, *Swine Influenza Immunization Program*, March 24, 1976.

INDEX

ABC News, 21, 102
ACIP (Advisory Committee on
Immunization Practices), 22,
25, 28–29, 35, 48, 65, 100,
230, 252
Alabama, Guillain-Barré syndrome
in, 96
Alaska, immunization stopped in,
91
Alexander, Russell, 27–28, 44, 60–
61, 68–69, 118
Allegheny County Health Department, 91–93
amantadine, 145–46, 229
American Insurance Association
(AIA), 70, 78–79
antibiotics, complications prevented by, 25, 255
antibodies, 146, 149–50, 228
Anti-Deficiency Act, 75, 82
antigenic shift:
influenza treatment hampered
by, 133–34, 149, 229–30
theory of, 18–19, 141–42,
144–45
antigens:
in vaccines, 148, 230
in viruses, 18, 141, 228
antiviral medication, 145–46

armed forces, U.S., immunization
plans for, 58, 147
Army, U.S.:
flu studied by, 21–22
vulnerability of recruits in,
23, 258
Asian flu, 18, 143, 145
Asiatic influenza, 143

Bangkok flu, 228, 230
Barrett, St. John, 74–75, 79, 82,
261–62
Bateman, Nancy, 258
Beattie, Richard, 110
Bennett, Ivan, 101
BoB (Bureau of Biologics), 20, 22,
51, 57, 72, 73, 111, 148
Review Panel on Viral and
Rickettsial Vaccine of, 65
role of, 52, 63–64, 256
"body count mentality," 92–93

Califano, Joseph, 99–104, 120–22,
225–27
at National Immunization Conferences, 106–8
California, immunization program
of, 64, 227

About the Authors

RICHARD E. NEUSTADT, author of *Alliance Politics* and *Presidential Power*, is the Lucius N. Littauer Professor of Public Administration in the John F. Kennedy School of Government at Harvard. Professor Neustadt was a White House assistant to President Truman and a consultant to Presidents Kennedy and Johnson on problems of government organization and operation.

HARVEY V. FINEBERG is a Professor of Health Policy and Management at the Harvard School of Public Health. He holds an M.D. from the Harvard Medical School and a Ph.D. in Public Policy from the Kennedy School of Government. Dr. Fineberg was an Intermediate Junior Fellow in Harvard's Society of Fellows and is a member of the National Academy of Sciences' Institute of Medicine.

DAVID A. HAMBURG, Director of the Division of Health Policy Research and Education at Harvard University and Professor of Public Policy and Management, lives with his wife in Cambridge, Massachusetts.

4671-4
5-10